W9-BUU-968

What people are saying about *A Death Prolonged*

A Death Prolonged is a fictional, fast-paced portrayal of very real problems that health care professionals and patients face every day. End-of-life situations are poorly managed today, and Dr. Gordon suggests several measures that could lead to substantial change. He presents a compelling case for the need to reallocate many health care dollars, spent ineffectively at the end of life, to far more-effective prevention and treatment options.

Charles A. Bush, M.D., Medical Director
The Ohio State University, Richard M. Ross Heart Hospital
Professor of Internal Medicine, Cardiovascular Medicine

I read it in one sitting. A gripping story of a young doctor's first-hand encounter with a deeply personal decision about death and the high price she paid. Jeff Gordon is a physician who has been there many times. This book explores the ethical and moral dimensions of life and death without being preachy. Few books portray the end-of-life ethical drama with such accuracy, sensitivity, and character development; this one is by far the best I've read.

Roger Brucker, Author of *The Longest Cave*,
Trapped! The Story of Floyd Collins, and other books

Dr. Jeff Gordon understands the value of communication and education among health care professionals, patients, and family/surrogate to address end-of-life care. The unique skills needed for this type of care are taught primarily at the bedside, but this book provides a platform for learning in an academic setting. *A Death Prolonged* should be mandatory reading for all students in health care professions, including pharmacy, nursing, and medicine.

Warren L. Wheeler, M.D., Medical Director, Palliative Medicine
Nathan Adelson Hospice, Las Vegas, Nevada

Within this intensely riveting story are the shocking truths about the state of end-of-life care in our country. You won't want to put this down, and you won't feel the same when you are finished.

Peter A. Accetta, M.D., Pathologist, Columbus, Ohio

A gripping story about a topic few of us think about, yet all of us need to address. A must read for all doctors involved in end-of-life care.

Jeffrey J. Barrows, D.O., M.A. (Bioethics), Health Consultant
Human Trafficking, Christian Medical Dental Association

Pastors need to read this book! No pat answers to difficult ethical issues—but an urgent plea to help people make good "end-of-life" decisions before they find themselves unable to do so. I hope Dr. Gordon's book gets the wide reading it deserves.

Gary DeLashmutt, Senior Pastor, Xenos Christian Fellowship

In a thrilling story, Dr. Gordon tackles a timely and difficult issue in a format that provides life-like situations we see every day. Patients, families, and physicians need the information this book provides, so they can make rational end-of-life decisions. Unfortunately, these discussions get put off and then when patients face life-ending illness or injury, neither they nor their families are prepared. This book provides a primer that will prepare people for the end of life before crisis strikes. The issue is real and is crippling health care. Our society cannot afford to ignore this matter.

Victoria Ruff, M.D., Director, Intensive Care Unit
Riverside Methodist Hospital, Columbus, Ohio

I am shocked that I had never even heard about this crucial issue. After finishing this book, I headed straight for my parents' house to talk to them. They were just as surprised by the facts as I was. But they were also relieved to get the chance to add a Do Not Resuscitate order to their living will before it was too late.

Jenny Hale, Teacher and Daughter

A Death Prolonged demonstrates that we, as physicians, can do more to effectively prepare our patients for their final days. It is a must read by physicians and patients.

Dhruti A. Suchak, M.D., Hospitalist, Grant Medical Center

As a nurse, I've agonized and grieved with patients and families. As a cancer patient, this book made me thankful that I have talked with my family, friends, doctors, and attorney about my wishes for end-of-life care, so I can avoid the pitfalls described in *A Death Prolonged*. This book will make you think about life.

Jill D. Steuer, Ph.D., R.N., C.N.S., Grant Medical Center

Practicing the truths put forward in this book will increase quality of health care and dramatically decrease health care costs.

Charlette Gallagher-Allred, Ph.D., R.D., L.D.
Co-author, *Taking the Fear Out of Eating*

A Death Prolonged

By
Jeff Gordon, M.D.

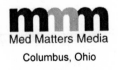

Med Matters Media

Columbus, Ohio

The views expressed in *A Death Prolonged* are those of the author and do not necessarily represent the views of Grant Medical Center or The Ohio State University College of Medicine and Public Health.

This publication is designed to provide accurate information regarding the material covered, but is not meant to render professional or legal advice or services. Please seek the counsel of the appropriate professional for these services.

Copyright © 2009 by Jeff Gordon, M.D.
All rights reserved. No part of this book may be reproduced or transmitted in any form or by any means, electronic or mechanical, including photocopying, recording, or by any information storage and retrieval system, without permission in writing from the publisher.

Published by Med Matters Media, LLC, Columbus, Ohio.
www.medmattersmedia.com

Printed in the United States of America

International Standard Book Number: 978-0-9819818-0-2

Cover art and design by David Groff
www.Groffillustration.com

Contents

For my wife, Laura,
and my children
Chris, Megan and Kate.

Introduction

Most Americans don't talk about dying. When they do, most are misinformed about what happens to people at the end of life. That's because most people get their information from television, and the TV fantasy world has created a level of ignorance that is hard to exaggerate. The dollar and human costs of this gross misinformation are astronomical. Many terminal patients linger through their final months with a miserable quality of life and too often with extreme levels of suffering. Today's high-tech medical care can sustain technical life—the beating heart—but utterly fails to restore real quality of life for many. The result: Death Prolonged.

Patients and loved ones need to know that they can choose treatment goals which allow a dignified natural death with minimal suffering, rather than a prolonged agonizing existence. Without intervention, millions of people face a lengthy, painful death over the next several years, and billions of precious health care dollars will be wasted. I'm committed to do what I can to prevent this.

This story is an attempt to tell the truth about end-of-life care in America. I chose fiction because people need more than facts: they need to *feel* these realities to get an accurate perspective.

This story is as close as I can come to taking you into the hospital, so you can experience these disturbing truths with me.

Every fact and statistic quoted in the story is real. The Source Notes on page 167 list all references by page of appearance.

You can get the most up-to-date information on these matters at **www.eoleducation.org**.

Jeff Gordon, M.D.
Grant Medical Center
Columbus, Ohio

*Facts are stubborn things; and whatever may be our wishes,
our inclinations, or the dictates of our passion,
they cannot alter the state of facts and evidence.*

John Adams
Argument in Defense of British Soldiers
in the Boston Massacre Trials

1

When Dr. Kate Simon strolled into the Emergency Department, three security guards were struggling to wrestle a roaring behemoth into leather restraints. They were outnumbered because his four extremities were like sprawling red oak branches and his massive hit of methamphetamine energized him beyond belief. He grunted and growled like an angry grizzly as they grappled him into the bed. Finally two hefty aides jumped into the fray to even the odds. Kate had seen some wild incidents in her first two weeks at Mercy Medical Center, but this fight was spectacular. A whopping man with a potent stimulant brewed a dangerous concoction.

Thanks to reinforcements, the guards restrained the crazed man on his back, one limb at a time. They battled to surround each wrist and ankle with padded leather straps, which they belted to the bed. One of the aides took a right hook to his face and ended up a patient himself with a broken nose. Once they finally laid him spread-eagle, a nurse rushed in, plunged a needle into his shoulder, and injected a sedative. He continued to glare and swear at his adversaries and tug at the belts. His drug-induced panic obscured all sensation of pain. After about 10 minutes, his neck finally relaxed, and his head fell back on the pillow. He was quiet at last.

The emergency room physician, Dr. Tom Garbella, glanced over his spectacles and said, "You'll be glad to know that gentleman won't be your patient, Dr. Simon. Yours is in Room 55. He's an elderly nursing home patient with a fever. Looks like he has a urinary-tract infection. You'd better get to work. They told me his blood pressure was dropping."

Kate felt relief knowing that another poor intern would get the brawler, but the other patient sounded pretty sick. She hurried down the hall, grabbed his chart, and scanned it to evaluate the lab results. She found the patient, Mr. Randal Jamis, had a high white blood-cell count and bacteria in his urine. Both were indicators of a urinary tract infection that most likely had spread to his blood stream. Next she surveyed his vital signs: heart rate, respirations, temperature, and blood pressure. Over the past two hours, his blood pressure had declined from 148/72 to 94/55, and his heart rate had gone from 92 to 133. He had a fever with a temperature of 101.8. All these signs were bad. Kate's pulse increased, too.

Without delay, Kate scurried in to see Mr. Jamis. One look and she knew he was sick. He was pale and sweating profusely. His respirations were rapid and shallow. Kate swallowed hard, grabbed her cell phone, and rang her senior resident, Dr. Jerome Jordan—J.J.

Her voice was calm and efficient. "Hey J.J., we've got a sick one. Could you come down and give me a hand?"

"What's up?" J.J. must have been catching a few winks. His voice was hoarse.

"We've got a 77-year-old gentleman who looks septic and he might be slipping into shock. His blood pressure's down to around 90, and his heart rate's up to 135."

J.J. perked up after hearing those numbers and asked, "Are you giving him fluids?"

"Fluids are running at about 150cc an hour."

"C'mon. That's like pissing in the ocean. He needs fluid, Simon. Start a 1000cc bolus of normal saline and run it wide open. I'll be right down." He paused, but before he closed his phone he commanded, "If he hasn't gotten antibiotics, get them ordered stat."

Kate understood the gravity of Mr. Jamis' situation. Overwhelming infections can cause extreme drops in blood pressure, creating septic shock. Blood pressure drops as blood vessels relax and dilate. The heart rate increases to compensate. Mr. Jamis was headed toward septic shock.

She also knew prompt intervention could save his life. Intravenous fluids expand the blood volume and increase blood pressure. Antibiotics fight off the organisms that cause infections. Since Mr. Jamis was a nursing home resident, powerful antibiotics were needed to fight off potentially resistant bacteria that flourish in health care settings. Kate called the hospital pharmacy and had the drugs sent up immediately.

After giving the order for the fluid infusion, Kate returned to the chart for a thorough review. Mr. Jamis was delirious and couldn't speak, so she had to rely on the chart.

J.J. arrived before the 1000cc of saline was in and marched straight to the bedside. He reviewed the vital signs, surveyed the situation, and asked Kate, "Any other data?"

"He's been a nursing home resident for the last four months since having a stroke. He can't walk but still eats; he conversed until he became ill. Today they noticed a decline in his alertness and called the squad."

"Any other medical history?"

"He has hypertension, prostate cancer, arthritis, besides the stroke I told you about."

"Okay, Simon. While I look this fellow over, you call the nursing home and see if you can get any more information."

Kate left the room, and J.J. examined Mr. Jamis from head to toe. He listened carefully to his back and chest and probed meticulously over his abdomen. Mr. Jamis grimaced as J.J. pressed on his lower abdomen. After completing his exam, he left to join Kate at the desk. J.J. studied the lab values and pulled Mr. Jamis' X-rays up on the computer.

When Kate finished on the phone, he asked, "Any more info?"

"The nurse said he's been having fevers off and on over the past four weeks. They've treated him for recurrent urinary tract infections. She said he develops fevers after he's been off the antibiotics for a few days. Other than that, the rest of the story's the same."

"It still sounds like a urinary tract infection with an organism that's resistant to the drugs they've prescribed." J.J. paused and added, "Let's be sure we get blood cultures before we start the antibiotics."

Kate nodded and with a hint of a smile said, "I got the cultures already."

"Good work," J.J. said. "Now examine him thoroughly and we'll discuss the case." He looked at the monitor and said, "His blood pressure is improving with the fluid bolus. We're headed in the right direction."

As Kate walked back into Mr. Jamis' room, she was thinking about those fevers, and she began looking for other causes of intermittent fevers. She combed carefully through the exam and stared at his hands and nails. She saw thin, dark discolorations like splinters beneath two nails on his right hand. Her pulse quickened and her eyes widened. She'd read about these and remembered pictures in a textbook, but she'd never seen a splinter hemorrhage before. Immediately she went to the heart exam. She listened carefully and could hear a blowing sound along the right side of the sternum. She could hear the sound radiate into the arteries in his neck.

When Kate walked out, J.J. had his feet propped up on the desk as he talked to another intern. He listened carefully and asked several questions as he guided another green doctor through a treatment decision. Kate started scribbling her note. After J.J. finished, he asked, "What do you think?"

"What'd you think of his murmur?" Kate asked.

J.J. shrugged. "I heard it. It wasn't very loud. It's probably just an old, stiff aortic valve."

"I guess it could be, but did you notice those splinter hemorrhages?" Kate said with measured excitement.

J.J.'s feet dropped like a stone. He jumped up and asked, "Splinter hemorrhages?"

"I think I found two on his right hand."

J.J. rushed into Room 55 and grabbed Mr. Jamis' hand. He stared at the nails, then grabbed the other hand. Without dropping the hand, he spun toward Kate. He had a big grin and his eyes twinkled. He practically shouted, "Dr. Simon, this is a great pick up. I missed these. You're not supposed to show up your senior resident—especially in your first month as an intern."

J.J. turned back toward Mr. Jamis and looked at the palms. Then he pulled down the lower eyelids and scrutinized every square millimeter. He whipped around, and with excitement growing in his voice, he said, "Look here: more evidence! See those little red spots on the lid? Those are hemorrhages, too, and most likely related to endocarditis. Wow, I haven't seen one of these cases in a long time!" Kate looked with interest, but she already knew about the conjunctival hemorrhages. That was her next question for J.J.

They finished their evaluation and contacted their attending physician. She had just finished medical school, and J.J. was in his third year of post-medical school training. Both were learning Family Medicine. Although J.J. was a fully licensed physician, he still was training, so he called his attending physician, Dr. John Dawson, to review the case. Dr. Dawson agreed with their assessment and plans and would see the patient in a few hours on morning rounds. Mr. Jamis continued to improve with IV fluids and antibiotics—disaster averted, thanks to Kate's sharp eye.

2

Kate didn't get a wink of sleep that night. She met three other new patients after midnight. In her spare moments, she combed over medical literature to learn as much as she could about her patients' conditions.

The team of Kate, J.J., two other residents, and a medical student met their attending physician, Dr. Dawson, in the intensive care unit (ICU). Dr. Dawson was a Professor of Internal Medicine at the local university. His research in infectious diseases led to prominence, but his real love was teaching young doctors and caring for patients. He conducted rounds at his patients' bedsides, so his charges could witness his interactions with them and their families. Besides the science of medicine, he trained them in its art: something caught not taught.

Mr. Jamis was the first patient on their list, and Kate presented his case. She discussed his history, as well as findings on physical exam and test results. She put the case together artfully and concluded with a cohesive plan of attack.

Before Dr. Dawson could ask a question, J.J. interrupted. He looked at the other residents and the student, and with a sheepish grin said, "Dr. Simon scooped me on this one, guys. I missed the signs of endocarditis."

Kate smiled and looked down at Mr. Jamis. Dr. Dawson took up the questions next. His questions for Kate spanned the spectrum regarding endocarditis. Kate's sleepless night of reading and hard work paid off: she was about to cross the finish line with flying colors when the final question came.

"What's Mr. Jamis' Code status, Dr. Simon?"

Kate's mouth went dry. In her excitement over the endocarditis, she forgot to contact the nursing home or family to find out about Mr. Jamis' Code status. He was not alert enough to discuss the matter.

Their previous Code status discussions flashed through her mind. Their first day, Dr. Dawson discussed Code status. He reminded them that unless designated otherwise, all patients receive full resuscitative efforts if their heart stops. When a patient needs resuscitation, "Code Blue" is announced over the hospital public address system. The Code includes CPR and other potentially life-saving interventions. Some patients decide in advance that they do not want heroic measures. It is the doctor's responsibility to obtain that information, so people are not resuscitated against their will. In other cases, people need to understand the facts about resuscitation, so they can make informed decisions about Code status. For those who decline resuscitation, physicians write a clear order: Do Not Resuscitate or DNR. Code status represents the patient's wishes regarding end-of-life care.

"I'm sorry, Dr. Dawson. I didn't address his Code status." Kate bit her lip and looked down. Being a perfectionist is risky business. Before Dr. Dawson resumed, Kate stole a glance at J.J., who would not look her way.

Like a great coach correcting his star quarterback, Dr. Dawson said, "Code status is an issue that you can't forget or neglect!" He continued, "Most people don't talk about Code status until it's too late, and then they suffer needlessly. If Mr. Jamis would have arrested, then you would have tried to resuscitate him. We need to know his wishes.

"I've had a few cases where people with a DNR Code status were resuscitated because of poor communication. That's a disaster."

Kate asked, "What chance would Mr. Jamis have of surviving a resuscitation attempt?"

"Good question. There are many issues to consider in estimating a person's chance of surviving resuscitation and eventually being released from the hospital or survival to discharge."

Dr. Dawson continued, "Mr. Jamis has several factors that lower his chances of surviving resuscitation including his age, the infection, and other medical problems, and he's in the intensive care unit. Research shows survival to discharge from zero percent to around 10 percent at best in this type of situation. I'd estimate his chances of survival to discharge to be around five percent or less."

Kate blurted, "Are you kidding? I thought people did better than that."

"It's a misconception that most people have, including doctors. Only about a third of doctors know accurate survival rates after resuscitation."

J.J. asked, "Do you think patients understand how grim their chances are of surviving resuscitation?"

"Clearly not. Researchers found that most people over age 70 believe their chances of surviving resuscitation are about 50 percent, not five.

"They found that patients get most of their information about medical issues from TV where resuscitations are successful about 67 percent of the time. People in the real world are making these crucial decisions with an overwhelming level of misinformation."

Dr. Dawson's expression hardened, and his tone toughened. "Very few people know the truth about this one simple issue. Every day, people suffer needlessly due to failed resuscitation attempts. I don't want that to happen on our service."

They finished rounds, and Kate left Mercy at noon, completing her 30-hour shift. Dr. Dawson returned to the ICU later that day and met with Mr. Jamis' son, Donald.

After introducing himself, Dr. Dawson said, "I want to update you on your father's condition and discuss our plans."

Donald nodded and Dr. Dawson proceeded. "Your father most likely has bacterial endocarditis. It's an infection on one of his heart valves. Our cardiologist did an echocardiogram this morning that shows a small growth on one of his heart valves. Blood culture results are not back yet, but we expect those tests will confirm the diagnosis. Right now he's stable."

Dr. Dawson paused and waited for a response. Donald asked, "What caused this?"

"Your father's aortic valve, which comes out of the main pumping chamber, has calcium in it, which is common in elderly people. He's had frequent infections over the past several months, and his abnormal valve became infected."

"How will you treat it?"

"It depends on what organism we culture, but in any case he will need several weeks of antibiotics through the IV line."

"Will he have to stay in the hospital for that?"

"No. We can insert a special IV line that can stay in place throughout the course." Dr. Dawson hesitated and asked, "Would your father want to undergo this type of treatment?"

"I think he would. He's still able to get around in a wheelchair and enjoy conversations with his friends. He's not ready to quit."

"We're treating the infection and will proceed. Now, sir, have you discussed end-of-life decisions with your father's physician?"

"Yes, Doctor. Dad doesn't want any heroic measures if he dies. He's been real clear on that." He stopped and asked, "Didn't that information make its way to you?"

"No sir, it didn't. I'm sorry about that."

"How can that get missed?" he asked with more than a hint of irritation.

"It requires communication between the nursing home and the hospital. Apparently they didn't send the document. Our doctors on-call failed to get the information. They clearly fumbled the ball, and I apologize."

"How can we prevent this in the future?"

"I'll complete a form that you can sign, since you are his legal power of attorney for health care. Keep a copy with you and on his chart at the nursing home. We will keep it on record here. His status will be Do Not Resuscitate, but we will continue to provide medical interventions like the IV fluids and antibiotics. Of course, we'll keep him comfortable."

"That's fine, but your system is pitiful. I can see how this could get screwed up all the time." His irritation was growing.

"Our system is a bad one for sure, but it's the best we have right now. We need a national database that lists people's end-of-life decisions. Then hospitals and emergency medical workers could treat them according to their decisions. It's a horrible mistake to resuscitate someone who asked to be left alone."

"That's worse than horrible. Don't let that happen to my dad."

Dr. Dawson sighed and said, "We'll do our best, sir. Do you have any other questions?"

"No, sir."

Dr. Dawson shook his head as he left the room, considering the distinct possibility that Mr. Jamis could have been coded that morning. He turned to the nurse who had followed him from the room and said, "He's right. Our system is pitiful. Things need to change."

3

When Kate entered Mercy three days later, she had her call bag slung over her shoulder. She felt rested and was ready for another 30-hour stint. She went straight to the ICU and found Mr. Jamis wide awake. His vital signs were stable, and they had identified the bacteria that caused the endocarditis. He'd be ready for discharge in a day or two with six weeks of IV antibiotics. The day blew by, and Kate prepared for another night on call.

The on-call shift began at 6 p.m. after residents finished a 12-hour day of work in the hospital or office. They covered the ER and took calls from nurses about patients on the floor. Kate and her fellow first-year residents or interns took the initial calls. The second- and third-year residents like J.J. provided guidance and helped the interns in tough situations. Attending physicians were available around the clock for consultation, and some spent the night in the hospital. Residents were required to leave the hospital by noon the following day, completing the 30-hour shift. Sometimes they slept; most of the time they didn't.

Between calls to evaluate patients in the ER and queries from floor nurses, interns didn't get much sleep or time to do much besides work. Most nights brought a steady stream of patients through the ER. Despite these vital duties, one call trumped them all: *Code Blue*—the clarion call for emergency resuscitation. At Mercy, three tones, *ping, ping, ping,* preceded the operator's overhead page: *Code Blue Room 822.*

The *ping, ping, ping* produced an adrenaline rush for Kate. As a medical student, she watched codes, but now she was a player. She sprinted to the codes, so she could do one of the key procedures, such as intubating or putting in a central line.

When someone is found unresponsive, resuscitation begins with the ABCs: airway, breathing, circulation. First ensure the airway is open by moving the head and jaw, then check for breathing and finally for a pulse. No breathing, no pulse—call the Code and start CPR.

Immediate delivery of oxygen to vital organs is crucial to successful resuscitation. A victim may suffer irreversible brain damage with only five minutes of oxygen deprivation. That's why Code Blue is an ultimate emergency. Code team doctors drop everything and bolt. The first person on the scene begins basic life support with CPR, and as others arrive, important procedures unfold.

Kate's Code Blue experience was growing rapidly, and that night on call would provide more opportunities to learn. Her first patient in the ER was Jerry Sebring, who presented with chest pain. He was a 42-year-old husband and father of three beautiful little girls. Jerry kept busy running his small construction company. He built houses and small commercial buildings.

Jerry greeted Kate with a smile and extended his thick hand. His wife Susan sat close by. Jerry began, "You look too young to be a doctor."

Kate heard that often. Looking at her blonde hair, blue eyes, and slender form caused most people to think of her as a college student, not a doctor. Their mistake became obvious after a brief conversation.

Kate returned the smile and said, "I'm Dr. Simon, one of the interns here at Mercy. I need to talk to you and examine you so we can get you admitted. What's the main reason you came in tonight?"

His smile evaporated, and with a deadpan expression he said, "My wife." She rolled her eyes and gave a hint of a scowl. Jerry broke into a grin and said, "Okay, I've been having chest pains."

"What's the pain feel like?"

"It's a pressure sensation."

"How long does it last?"

"About two to five minutes. It depends…"

"Depends on what?" asked Kate.

"Depends on what I'm doing."

"What brings it on?"

"If I'm lifting or hammering—stuff like that."

"What caused it today?"

"I was digging a ditch in our yard, and it started. I sat down, and the pain was about gone when my wife came out. And here we are. She nagged me into this. I think it's just a little heartburn."

"It might be heartburn, but it could be your heart." Kate continued the questions. "How long have you been having this pain?"

"Off and on for about three or four weeks."

"Do you have any other problems when you have the pain?"

Jerry thought for several seconds and looked away. Then he nodded his head and said, "Yeah, sometimes I get a little sweaty, and I've had some nausea, too. That's why I think it's heartburn."

"Mr. Sebring, your story is extremely concerning for heart pain. The ER doctor started you on the medication protocol we use in cases where someone is threatening a heart attack. Right now your EKG, which shows electrical activity in your heart, is normal, and you have no evidence of a heart attack on your lab tests, but we need to observe you closely and get some other tests."

"What tests will I need?"

"I need to confer with my supervising resident, and we'll be in touch with a heart specialist, a cardiologist, tonight, so he knows about your situation. He will decide which other tests you need. His name is Dr. Fishman."

Kate saw Mrs. Sebring's eyes well with tears. She took a few steps toward her and said, "You did the right thing by getting him in here. There's no evidence of a heart attack, and we'll keep a close watch on him. He's not going anywhere until we get this all figured out."

Mrs. Sebring wiped her eyes, sniffled, and with a quivering voice said, "Thank you, Dr. Simon. I appreciate everything that you've done for Jerry."

"We'll take good care of him."

Kate finished her interview and examined him carefully. His exam and tests were normal; his story was ominous. That's why Kate and J.J. admitted Jerry to one of the cardiac beds with EKG monitoring. Kate checked on him later that evening. He was watching a baseball game and sipping a cup of decaffeinated coffee, which he deplored. No caffeine on the cardiac diet. He told Kate what he really wanted was an ice cold beer.

About an hour later, Kate's cell phone buzzed. The nurse's voice was pressured. "Mr. Sebring in Room 6005 started having chest pain. He's short of breath, pale, and sweating profusely. I gave him a Nitro. Can you come and see him now?"

"I'm on my way."

Kate bolted for the elevator and called J.J. for backup. This situation could be bad. Jerry was having a heart attack. While waiting at the elevator, she heard *ping, ping, ping...Code Blue Room 6005.* Oh, no! Jerry was coding!

Kate, J.J., and the rest of the Code team arrived immediately. Nurses were performing CPR. Jerry did not look like the vigorous young father of three she had just left, as the nurse pumped up and down on his chest. Jerry had been on an EKG monitor, and they immediately recognized the potentially fatal, but treatable, heart rhythm called ventricular fibrillation.

"Charge the defibrillator to 360 joules and defibrillate!" shouted J.J. The nurse handed the paddles to Kate, who was at the bedside. Her eyes darted toward each paddle. She had shocked a dummy, but never a man. She remembered the protocol and performed it precisely. Place one paddle at the bottom and the other at the top of the heart, yell "All clear!" and squeeze both buttons. She watched Jerry's muscles contract as the current coursed through his body on the way to his heart. Then she looked to the monitor along with every set of eyes in the room. The line went flat for two or three seconds then blip, blip, blip: normal sinus rhythm.

J.J. separated the crowd and pushed his hand into Jerry's groin area to check for a pulse in the femoral artery. Kate stared at J.J. for what seemed an eternity. He spun his head toward Kate and said, "He's got a pulse." He turned to the pharmacist. "We need a dose of amiodarone now." His eyes shot back to Kate. "Go call Dr. Fishman so he can take this guy to the cath lab." Next he turned to the nurses and said, "We need a 12-lead EKG."

J.J. kept his finger on the pulse for the next minute or so and felt it strengthen with each beat. Jerry began to stir and took a deep breath. The resuscitation was done so quickly that he did not get intubated. J.J. listened to his lungs and pressed on his chest, feeling for broken ribs.

The EKG confirmed their suspicions: a heart attack involving the front of his heart—an anterior myocardial infarction. The small blood vessel coursing down the front wall of Jerry's heart was blocked, and it was threatening to kill him.

By the time they started the amiodarone to prevent more ventricular fibrillation and wheeled Jerry to the catheterization lab, Dr. Fishman was ready with his team. He looked at the EKG, listened to Jerry's chest with his stethoscope, and said, "Mr. Sebring, you're having a heart attack. We need to perform a catheterization and open the artery if we can. Are you agreeable?"

Jerry was groggy but awake. He said, "Do what you need to do, Doc. I want to see my daughters again." He turned to Kate and asked, "Why's my chest hurt so bad?"

Kate grasped his hand and followed along as they wheeled Jerry into position. She said, "You're having a heart attack, and we just

resuscitated you. I'll explain it all later. You're doing okay right now."
She broke away as the cath lab team took over. Later she would
explain that the CPR and defibrillation—those life-saving
measures—come with a cost: a bruised sternum, sore ribs, and some
minor burns from the shock. It was a small price in exchange for his
life.

Dr. Fishman managed to open the artery with a tiny balloon-
tipped catheter and placed a metal stent across the area of blockage
to keep the vessel open. He found no other blockages. Jerry spent
the night under close observation in the ICU. He continued to
improve through the night and early morning hours.

Kate stopped by the ICU around 3 a.m. Jerry was sound asleep.
She stood in his doorway with her hands in the pockets of her white
lab coat. She looked at the monitor, and a satisfied smile grew as she
gazed at normal sinus rhythm. Her enthusiasm and marvel for
medicine reached an all-time high that morning, but her zeal for
resuscitation was about to be challenged.

Kate was finishing a note on the eighth floor around 5:30 a.m.
when she heard, *ping, ping, ping, Code Blue Room 8021.*

4

Kate was just down the hall from Room 8021. As she sprinted to the room, she swelled with anticipation, thinking about Jerry's great save.

Kate was the first doctor in Mrs. Angela Frank's room, followed by the respiratory therapist. She hurried to the bedside, and the nurse asked her to take over chest compressions. Kate had performed chest compressions several times and was gaining a feel for the technique. Moving her weight up and down on outstretched arms, she pressed firmly on the sternum with the heel of her hand, quickly bouncing up and down, to achieve 100 to 120 compressions each minute. By now, she knew what it was like to feel the chest move up and down under her hand—knowing that blood was flowing to vital organs.

CPR is ineffective if the compressions are too shallow. The sternum must move substantially under the weight of the compressions to squeeze the heart against the spine and move the blood forward. Kate was not timid with her compressions.

Kate knelt on the patient's bed at her right side. The back board was in place to brace Mrs. Frank against the pressure on her chest, so the compressive force would go into her chest and not just bury her in the bed. Kate identified the correct area, placed the heel of her hand on the naked sternum, positioned her shoulders over her outstretched arms, and pressed—just like always. She stopped after one compression, winced, and resumed CPR.

Kate had never felt bones shatter beneath her hands before. To hear the sickening crack of breaking ribs was something she never expected. As she moved up and down counting, "one, two, three, four...," the ribs and sternum played a horrible tune of their own, snapping with each compression. The rest of the Code team arrived, and the wild dance continued.

J.J. rushed into the room and bolted to the head of the bed. He popped off the headboard while he asked for the laryngoscope. The nurse handed him the silver scope with a curved blade, and in one smooth motion, he swept the tongue aside and lifted the jaw so he could see the two vocal cords, which mark the opening of the windpipe. He inserted the plastic endotracheal tube between the vocal cords and attached a bag-like device that he pressed on to drive air into her lungs. Immediately, another resident listened for breath sounds as the chest wall rose with each squeeze of the bag.

J.J. glanced at the monitor and noted her slow heart rhythm. He shouted through the chaos, "Half a milligram of atropine now, and get an amp of epinephrine ready to go." The pharmacist passed the syringe to Kate who pushed it into the IV line. The patient needed a second dose of each medication to increase her heart rate to an acceptable level. After about 12 minutes of chest compressions, Mrs. Frank was alive again—at least her heart was beating, and she had a pulse.

As they made arrangements for a transfer to the ICU, Kate studied Mrs. Frank. She was pale and extremely thin: cachectic. Kate could count every rib. Her eyes were sunken, and her cheek bones jutted out like an Auschwitz victim. Her spine curved forward, so her shoulders appeared hunched from the bone-thinning impact of osteoporosis. She was obviously chronically ill and undernourished.

J.J. asked, "Anyone know this patient?"

Ken Chan, one of Kate's fellow interns, spoke up. "I admitted her last night. The squad brought her in from the nursing home because she passed out."

"What's up with her mental status and nutrition? I haven't seen anyone this malnourished in a long time."

"I reviewed the records from the nursing home. She's been there for about a year, and she's had Alzheimer's disease for about three years. She knows her name and that's about it. Short-term memory is gone. She hasn't recognized her family members for about the last year. Her appetite's declined since she was treated for pneumonia here about a month ago. She passed out today, and they brought her in."

"Did you ask about Code status?"

"I looked all over the records and called the nursing home. As far as they knew, she's Full Code."

J.J. and Kate transferred Mrs. Frank to the ICU on a ventilator and called the cardiologist. They sat together at the desk in the center of the ICU, and finished some paperwork. No one had much to say.

Kate broke the silence. "Now I see why Dr. Dawson hounds us about Code status. I'll never forget the feel of those splitting ribs and sternum." She cringed and shuttered.

J.J. glanced up and said, "You'll get another chance, Simon." He looked back down and kept writing.

"You mean you've done this before?"

J.J. nodded and said, "Too many times to remember. I'd like to forget them all."

"That's mind-blowing, J.J." They were silent for several seconds, and then Kate asked, "What did we accomplish?"

"To use Dr. Dawson's words, we prolonged her dying. And we crushed her chest."

Kate sat silently. Her forehead glistened and dark circles were forming under her eyes. Her hair had become a tangled mass. She stared at the chart on the desk.

J.J. nudged her and put his hand on her shoulder. "Listen Kate, we're the Code team. We had no choice. She was a Full Code."

"You're right, but it still seems crazy." Kate hesitated and asked, "Do you think she's in pain?"

"She's moving her arms and legs, so I'd say she's in some pain, but we'll sedate her after we get her blood pressure up a little higher. Then she'll be pain free."

"Do you think she felt pain during the Code?"

"I'm not sure. She probably did. She had several rib fractures, and they're really painful."

"Do you think she'll recover, J.J.?"

"No way. Didn't you listen to Dr. Dawson? Her chances of recovery are slim to none. If against all odds she did recover to be discharged, what do you think her quality of life would be? Do you think anyone would want to live this way?"

"How long do you think she'll suffer like this?"

"I gave up trying to predict when someone will die. Maybe her family will be sensible and let her die naturally and in peace."

"I wonder if anyone discussed Code status with her or her family."

"I gave up trying to predict that too, but if you're a betting person, you'd bet on 'No' because most people have never had an end-of-life discussion with their doctor."

Kate sighed and shook her head. "This is maddening, J.J." She pushed her chair back and headed for the door. "I'm gonna check on that guy with the heart attack before rounds."

5

They met for rounds in the ICU. Dr. Dawson looked up as Kate, J.J., and Ken strolled into the unit. He nodded toward Jerry's room, and with a broad grin said, "Great save! Looks like he's doing well." He shook their hands to celebrate the victory like a proud father reveling in his son's winning touchdown. He turned and headed into Jerry's room.

Dr. Dawson introduced himself and reviewed Jerry's history. "How are you feeling?" he asked.

"I'm a little sore in the chest, and it feels like I have a burn right there," he said, pointing to the top area of his chest.

"The soreness is from the chest compressions. They did CPR to revive you last night," said Dr. Dawson as he gestured toward the team.

Jerry nodded and glanced through the room at each resident.

Dr. Dawson continued, "The small burn is from the machine they used to shock your heart back into rhythm." He hesitated and pointed to the team and with half a smile said, "Sorry about that, but it's the best they could do under the circumstances."

Jerry grinned and sat up straight. "No problem. I just wondered why I felt so sore."

"CPR is a vigorous procedure. To move the blood forward, we must depress the chest far enough to compress the heart, and that requires quite a push. You can imagine why you hurt."

Jerry nodded. "These doctors did a great job. I can't tell you how grateful I am."

"It sounds like you need to thank that nagging wife of yours, too. You might not be here if it weren't for her persistence."

Jerry chuckled and said, "You can bet I won't forget that...and neither will she." He paused and his face turned grim. He grabbed a photo of three beautiful little girls from his bedside table and turned back to the team. He dropped his head for a few seconds, and when he looked up, tears were in his eyes. "You'll never know how much I appreciate what you did for me last night." He pointed to each girl and said, "Those girls get their daddy back."

Kate and J.J. gave a subtle fist pump after clearing the door. Kate had not experienced a feeling of accomplishment like this since winning the Big Ten Conference cross-country title. This made the hard work and long hours worth the effort. They saved his life!

The mood changed as they walked into Mrs. Frank's room—like entering a musty cellar after a sunny day at the beach. A knot grew in Kate's stomach as she relived the resuscitation. She cringed as she thought about the broken bones and shivered watching the chest expand and contract under the ventilator's power. If not for the heavy sedatives, the pain would be excruciating, but Mrs. Frank didn't move. Kate was glad the sedatives worked.

Dr. Dawson stood in silence at her bedside and shook his head. He stared through the window and finally said, "This poor soul should not be treated this way. What happened, Ken?"

"I called the nursing home, and the charge nurse told me she was a Full Code. I left a message with her family, but no one called back. I don't think anyone has ever discussed Code status with the patient or her family."

Dr. Dawson's head continued to shake. He turned to Ken and said, "You did everything you could."

He examined her and said, "I think she's well sedated and pain free. Get her family in here ASAP, so we can confer with them and decide how to proceed. I can't imagine they'd want to prolong her dying."

6

Mrs. Frank's only daughter, Julie Kingston, lived in town and came to Mercy that morning to meet with Dr. Dawson and the team. They met at Mrs. Frank's bedside. Dr. Dawson filled her in on the events of the evening, including the resuscitation. He also reviewed Mrs. Frank's story and confirmed some key details, including the fact that her condition had been steadily declining over the past year.

Dr. Dawson asked, "Does she remember her name?"

"She knows her name, but she can't remember me or any of her friends." A tear welled in Mrs. Kingston's eye, and she whisked it away.

"Will she talk with you?"

"No," Mrs. Kingston whispered and looked down.

"Has she been agitated or confused?"

"She's been increasingly angry, and last week she struck a nurse."

"Is her condition stable or declining in your opinion?"

"She's getting worse every day," said Mrs. Kingston, as she sighed deeply.

"Has anyone discussed end-of-life issues with you and your mother?"

"What do you mean?"

"People have choices when it comes to medical treatment. Many people who are elderly and have failing health decline medical treatments that would prolong their lives."

She frowned and asked, "Why do people refuse medical treatment?"

"That decision usually comes when their quality of life is poor. For example, if a person can't do the things that make them happy and they are suffering, they might decide to stop medical therapies that would prolong their lives. There comes a point when physicians can prolong dying, but not provide quality living. It's a personal choice."

She paused and her expression hardened. Then she demanded, "Do you mean doctors just let people die?"

"Mrs. Kingston, this is a choice that patients and their families make. No doubt it's difficult and every situation is different, but some people decide against medical treatments that extend life and seek Comfort Care only."

"Does that mean that you kill them?"

"No, we don't speed their death. We treat their pain and anything that might cause discomfort and let nature take its course. Instead of prolonging their death, we let them die in peace."

Some of the tension eased from her face. "Are you saying that instead of treating my mom's medical problems, we treat her pain and let her die naturally?"

"That's one choice: Comfort Care only."

"What would you recommend, Dr. Dawson?"

"I'd recommend Comfort Care only, Mrs. Kingston."

"Why not treat her medical conditions?"

"Your mother's health is poor and declining. Her nutrition is terrible, which makes it practically impossible for her to heal. She would probably spend the rest of her life on the ventilator. Besides that, her quality of life before this resuscitation was not good. It's highly unlikely that she will recover—even if we do everything in our power."

Her eyes filled and her voice wavered. "Do you think it's hopeless?"

"There's practically no hope of recovery, but we can provide Comfort Care and let her die in peace with dignity."

Mrs. Kingston sat silently, seemingly mesmerized by the whirl of the ventilator.

Dr. Dawson broke the silence. "What do you think your mom would want?"

She wiped her eyes and took a deep breath. "We didn't discuss it exactly, but I remember her comments about a friend's situation. Her friend was hospitalized and ended up on a ventilator for a long time. Mom said that she didn't want to be kept alive by machines." She hesitated and looked down. "I wish we would have discussed these issues when she was lucid," she said, as tears rolled down her face. She looked back up and said, "What should we do now?"

"Here are the options. One option is to continue the full level of support. We call that Full Code. That's her status now. If her heart stops again, we would resuscitate her again."

Mrs. Kingston interrupted, "I don't want her to go through that again. What are the other options?"

"Another option is to change her status to Do Not Resuscitate. Then we would continue the present level of care, but we would not try to resuscitate her if her heart stops. That's what we call DNR with medical intervention." He paused to allow a question.

"Then she would remain on the breathing machine, right?"

"That's correct."

"What else would you do?"

"She would probably need a pacemaker to treat the abnormal heart rhythm."

"Are there other options?"

"The third option is to provide Comfort Care only. We would keep your mother comfortable and stop treatments that prolong her life."

"Would that include the breathing machine?"

"Yes," Dr. Dawson nodded.

Mrs. Kingston looked at her mom, unresponsive on the ventilator. Tears continued to stream down her cheeks. "Doctor, I don't want my mom to suffer, but I don't want to kill her."

"First of all, to withhold life-prolonging medical treatments and let her die naturally is not killing her. We would keep her comfortable through the whole process and do nothing to deliberately speed her death. Neither the DNR nor the Comfort Care option is killing her."

"What would you do, Dr. Dawson?"

"I think her death will come soon no matter what we do. At this point, we are prolonging her death. If I were you, I'd opt for Comfort Care."

There was a long silence.

Dr. Dawson resumed, "I know this is a lot to think about. You don't need to decide right now."

He waited for Mrs. Kingston to respond, but she said nothing. "Is there someone you can talk to, like your pastor or a close friend?"

Her expression relaxed, and she said, "That's a good idea. I need time to think this over, and discussing it with my pastor is a good idea."

"We'll stop back later today to see if you have any questions," said Dr. Dawson, as he shook her hand and left the room.

As they left her room, Dr. Dawson turned to the team and said, "I'm glad she's speaking with her pastor today. Some pastors are more attentive to end-of-life discussions than we are."

As they walked to the next room, Kate could not have imagined the impact this next young patient would have on her future.

Toni Jackson was a 22-year-old student at the local community college. She had been treated for diabetes since she was 14 and was admitted to Mercy with Diabetic Ketoacidosis or DKA. This life-threatening illness develops in diabetics who are deficient in insulin and encounter circumstances that produce an increase in stress hormones. Typical stressors include intestinal viruses, infections, and heart attacks. Some diabetics develop DKA if they stop taking their insulin.

Toni was in DKA because she was broke and ran out of insulin. She was struggling to make ends meet while working full time and going to school. Her income was too high to get government assistance, so she lived among the ranks of the uninsured. She made it to the last week of the month and ran out of money and insulin at the same time. She was in DKA simply because she was poor. She would gladly take her insulin if she had it.

Toni felt much better thanks to Kate's excellent care and the wonders of IV insulin and IV fluids. Her heart rate was down; blood pressure was normal; nausea and breathlessness were gone.

Dr. Dawson reviewed her story and examined her. He turned to Toni and said, "Looks like you've done quite well."

Toni looked across the room at Kate and said, "Thanks to Dr. Simon. I guess I was sicker than I thought."

Kate smiled with the growing satisfaction of another save.

Toni looked at the team of physicians, then around the ICU with all its gadgets and fell silent. She paused for several seconds, lost in turmoil, then asked with panic in her voice, "How much will all this cost?"

Her question took the whole team off guard. Kate had not considered the issue of cost in Toni's case. She focused on treating patients and let others worry about that stuff, so Toni's question was new.

Her question even knocked Dr. Dawson off balance. In an uncertain tone, he said, "Well…I'm not sure, Ms. Jackson."

Toni's tone was intense. "I need to know because I don't have insurance and I'm barely getting by. I'm here because I ran out of money and couldn't buy my insulin. It's about $40 a vial. I know I can't miss a dose, but I ran out of money…" Toni trailed off and looked away.

"We have social workers and financial counselors that can help you. For now, focus on getting better. Worry about the bill later." His response lacked his typical confidence.

Toni looked down and covered her face in an unsuccessful attempt to hide her tears and embarrassment. She sniffed and wiped her eyes. "It's hard for me *not* to worry, Dr. Dawson, with all my bills."

"We'll have our social worker see you and help you figure it out. Who is your doctor, so we can arrange follow up?"

"I don't have a doctor. I go to the free clinic on Second Street, but I don't go very often because I have to wait forever. I can't afford the wasted time."

Kate interrupted, "Toni's schedule is more demanding than ours, Dr. Dawson. When she's not in class, she's working or studying. Is there any way we could help her?"

Dr. Dawson looked back at Toni. "You can see Dr. Simon in our clinic that's right across the street. Mercy operates the clinic, and we take care of uninsured patients. Would that work?"

Kate looked surprised. She'd forgotten that she was scheduled to begin seeing patients in the clinic.

Toni's apprehension persisted, and she asked, "How long will I have to wait?"

Kate chimed in, "I'll be on time, so don't worry about that."

Toni swept her tears away, and a smile of relief grew across her face. "I'd love to have Dr. Simon as my doctor."

It was settled. Toni would see Kate in the Mercy Clinic. Kate was eager to do what she could to help Toni stay healthy.

The team finished their rounds on the floor and returned to the ICU to meet with Mrs. Kingston. Kate hoped they would be able to answer her questions and do what was best for Mrs. Frank.

When Dr. Dawson came to the doorway, Mrs. Kingston was sitting at her mother's bedside, caressing her thin pale hand and stroking her face. Her pastor, Henry Heintzman, a tall, athletic-looking man in a polo shirt and khakis, stood beside her.

The ventilator whined softly in the background, and every four seconds a whoosh of air signaled another mechanical breath. Her chest rose and fell, signaling the completion of another cycle. The plastic endotracheal tube protruded from the right side of her open mouth. A piece of tape circuited her cheeks and neck to secure the tube. Another plastic tube ran from her left nostril to her stomach. This nasogastric tube decompressed and emptied the stomach after a code and could be used for nutrition.

Another tube, the urinary catheter, emptied the bladder. A balloon at its tip kept it in place, maintaining a constant flow of urine. Her last tubes were two IV lines—one in each arm. Five adhesive patches about two centimeters square secured wires for monitoring her EKG. A plastic clip with a red light clung to her index finger, monitoring blood oxygen levels.

A plastic blood pressure cuff attached to her right upper arm by way of Velcro automatically inflated and deflated to measure blood pressures periodically. Above her was a 17-inch LCD display of the vital information.

Dr. Dawson hesitated in the doorway to survey the scene. He looked at each piece of high-tech equipment and then at the victim in her bed.

He knocked on the door frame. Pastor Heintzman and Mrs. Kingston turned, and she said, "Dr. Dawson, please come in."

He nodded and asked, "Is she comfortable?"

"I think so. The nurses have done a good job. The medications keep her sedated, and she seems to feel no pain." She grasped her mother's hand more tightly and with pleading eyes asked, "Do you think she's in pain?"

Dr. Dawson walked to the other side of the bed, listened to her chest with his stethoscope, felt the mangled rib cage and sternum, as he watched for a grimace. He probed her abdomen and moved her legs. Then he said, "She's comfortable."

"Can she feel pain?"

"Right now she is sedated, so she doesn't choke on the breathing tube or feel pain, particularly in her chest."

"Why would she have chest pain?" Mrs. Kingston asked with growing concern.

"When the doctors performed chest compressions to resuscitate her, they broke several ribs and possibly her breast bone. I'm sorry, but in frail people like your mother, broken ribs are common with resuscitation." His voice remained calm and reassuring.

She sighed and asked, "Can she hear me?"

"I'm not sure, but go ahead and talk to her. That might soothe her. We'll do everything we can to keep her pain free."

Mrs. Kingston looked at her pastor, then back to Dr. Dawson and said, "Pastor Heintzman and I have been talking about Mom's Code status. I wish Mom and I would have talked while she was still sharp. I feel like I let her down, but I didn't want to bring up the issue of death with her. I was afraid I'd discourage her or make her think I was ready to get rid of her." She dropped her head.

Dr. Dawson moved to her side. "Unfortunately, lots of people find themselves in your exact situation, but we can work together to get the best outcome for your mom."

The reassurance brought a hint of relief to Mrs. Kingston's face.

Dr. Dawson continued, "Have you considered what your mother would want? Think about what she valued and lived for."

"That's what Pastor Heintzman and I have been talking about. We agree that she wouldn't want to live this way. What you said struck me—now we're prolonging her dying, not helping her live. She's lived a good life, and I remember her saying, 'I'd rather live a good life than a long life.'"

Mrs. Kingston continued, "You know, Dr. Dawson, she has not had a good life for a long time. Mom's been deteriorating for months in the nursing home. She's been in and out of the hospital several times, and each time was painful. Then last night she had her chest broken with that resuscitation, and look at her now." She stopped and wiped her eyes. The pastor put his hand on Mrs. Kingston's shoulder.

She took a deep breath and pressed on. "Mom would not want to live this way. I feel bad because I don't think she would have wanted to live the way she has for the past two years. I wish I would have talked to her doctor."

"I'm sorry, Mrs. Kingston. Sometimes the medical system fails people like your mother. We need to focus on what's best for her now. What do you want us to do?"

She pointed to the ventilator and the tubes. "I'm certain that Mom would not want this. I don't want her to continue to suffer with no hope of recovery. Please keep her comfortable, but stop these machines. I want her to be at peace."

"Do you mean stop the ventilator?" asked Dr. Dawson.

"Yes. But only if we know she will be comfortable."

"We will definitely keep her comfortable. We will provide medications that will take away any feeling of breathlessness. She will not feel pain."

"But will we be killing her?" Mrs. Kingston asked again with apprehension.

"No, we will not," declared Dr. Dawson emphatically. "We will allow her to die a natural death. We will take no steps to cause her death."

Mrs. Kingston sighed, "Okay, I understand, but I can't get that idea out of my head."

"I understand your reservations, and I want you to know that withholding care is not causing a death. We allow her to die naturally. I want to be sure you grasp this because many people end up feeling guilty later if they don't appreciate the distinction. Do you understand?"

"I think so, Doctor. I know she did not want to live like this, so Comfort Care without the ventilator is the way I think we should go."

Pastor Heintzman squatted down and looked Mrs. Kingston straight in the eye and said, "You're making the right decision. I would do the same thing. I'm sorry that I didn't bring this up earlier."

Dr. Dawson put his hand on her shoulder. "I know how hard this must be. If I were in your situation, I'd make the same decision. We'll keep your mother comfortable."

"How soon will you stop the ventilator?"

"Are you ready now or would you like other friends or family here with you?" asked Dr. Dawson.

"If it's okay, I'd love for my son to be here. He's on his way and will be here in an hour or so."

"That's fine. Dr. Simon will check back with you, and when you're ready, we will go ahead and stop the breathing machine. Now in the meantime, I suggest we change her status to DNR, just in case her heart stops. From what you said, you would not want her put through resuscitation again."

"That's right," said Mrs. Kingston.

"So for now, your mom's status is DNR, and after your family is together, we will change that to Comfort Care and stop the ventilator. Is that what you want?"

"Yes."

"We'll write the orders and let the nurses know. They will call us when your family arrives. Do you have any other questions?"

"No, Dr. Dawson. Thank you so much for your kindness. I can't tell you how much I appreciate what you and your staff have done for me and my mom."

"I'm glad we could help you," said Dr. Dawson.

He shook her hand, but before he could leave, Pastor Heintzman asked, "Doctor, could I ask you a few questions outside before you leave?"

"Sure, Pastor."

They moved into the hall, and the pastor asked, "What could I do to prevent this in the future?"

"I'm glad you're interested, Pastor. This is a big problem, and people need help making end-of-life decisions. You and your fellow clergy could make a big impact because most people are completely uninformed on the issues."

"I must admit, I have a lot to learn. Where should I start?"

Dr. Dawson handed him his business card. "Give me a call and we'll get together."

"Thanks."

They shook hands, and Dr. Dawson led the team out of the ICU. They finished their work.

An hour later, Kate and Dr. Dawson returned to the ICU. They found Mrs. Kingston standing next to her son and Pastor Heintzman at the bedside. They had said their goodbyes and were ready to see their loved one's suffering end.

Dr. Dawson asked the nurse to administer a dose of sedative to ensure that Mrs. Frank would not feel breathless when the ventilator was stopped. A few minutes after the dose, the ventilator was disconnected from the plastic endotracheal tube. Mrs. Frank made shallow respiratory efforts, but there were no signs of panic or pain. After several minutes, the breathing pattern became erratic, and the blood pressure dropped precipitously. There were no signs of struggle as Mrs. Frank's breathing stopped after about 10 minutes. Her blood pressure continued to fall, and her heart rate declined as the nurse periodically checked her pulse. After about 20 minutes, the EKG was flat, respirations were absent, and she had no pulse. Mrs. Frank was at peace.

The nurse told her daughter that she had died. The finality of those words struck Mrs. Kingston like they do most people. Mrs. Kingston wept.

There was so much for Kate to think about. She'd been working for almost 30 hours, and her shift was done at noon. She was eager to get home, get some rest, and go for a run with her sister, Meg.

9

Kate's crisp sheets felt amazing. She set her alarm for 6 p.m. and shut off her cell phone. That would give her a four-hour nap. When the alarm buzzed, she didn't remember hitting the pillow. Climbing out of bed was like scaling a cliff. Her feet finally hit the floor as she rubbed her eyes while yawning. She sat on the bed as her head cleared, and she finally remembered that it was evening, not morning. She smiled, realizing that it was time for play and not work. Within a few minutes, she was jogging toward the park to meet Meg.

Shadows were lengthening, and the air was cooler thanks to an afternoon thunderstorm. Kate pounded through puddles, and steam rose from the sidewalk. She remembered her jogs through the streets of Phnom Penh, Cambodia, with her dad during the rainy season. She lived in Phnom Penh for 10 years while her parents operated a medical clinic, serving that crowded city's poorest people. She smiled as she thought about her parents, turned the corner, and saw Meg ahead.

Meg looked up as Kate arrived. "Hi, Kate. Any excitement last night?"

"You love these medical tales too much," Kate said. "You should have gone to med school."

Meg wrinkled her nose with a playful scowl. "You know I hate blood, and I can't stand to hear people gag and spit," she said, shivering.

"I'm still getting used to the spitting." They both laughed.

"Let's go. I'll tell you about the night while we run."

"Maybe that'll slow you down."

They took off into the park with Kate setting the pace and doing most of the talking. She told Meg about Jerry, Toni, and Mrs. Frank. By the time they reached the three-mile mark, Kate had told her about Mrs. Frank's death. They stopped to catch their breath.

Meg was puzzled. She wiped the sweat from her face. "I don't understand why you let that lady die after all those heroics."

"We talked to her daughter for a long time, and she knew that her mother would not want to be kept alive with the ventilator. Her mother's quality of life had been poor for a long time. She was certain that her mom would not want to have her death prolonged."

Kate stood by a bench and stretched her calves. "No one had discussed Code status with this lady's daughter before yesterday, and that's what created the problem."

"That's pitiful! This poor lady suffered through all that misery just because no one talked to her or her daughter about Code status."

Kate nodded, motioned to the path, and resumed their workout.

They ran through the park's sprawling rose garden and turned toward home.

Suddenly Meg said, "Stop, Kate."

"What's wrong, Meg?"

"Your first patient almost died because she couldn't get a $40 vial of insulin, right?"

"Yeah."

"She's young, uninsured, and poor?"

"Yeah."

"How many of those $40 vials of insulin does she need?"

"About one and a half a month."

"That's $60 a month." Meg wiped her face. "It sounds to me like the resuscitation of that other patient was unnecessary."

"We had to do it. She was a Full Code."

"I know you *had* to do it," said Meg. "It was unnecessary in the sense that a conversation between the family and her doctor could have prevented that resuscitation. Right?"

"Absolutely."

"So how much do you think her hospitalization cost?"

Kate stood in silence for several seconds. "I don't know. It had to cost a lot. Probably thousands."

"What are the costs?"

Kate smiled and joked, "And now for a cost analysis by Meg Simon."

"Come on, humor me."

"All right, Meg. First of all, you have the emergency room costs, including blood tests, X-rays, nursing and physician care. Then hospital costs like medications, nurses and doctors, and everything it takes to operate the hospital.

"Then the Code Blue, including personnel, equipment, and more drugs. Finally, she was in the ICU, which is super expensive. It had to be thousands of dollars."

"You're saying thousands of dollars were spent on someone who didn't want medical care while this young woman can't get a $40 vial of insulin."

Kate was overwhelmed by the starkness of Meg's conclusion but could not refute it. She said, "That's right."

"I don't want to be crass," Meg said, "But you're saying that last night someone, I guess the government or the taxpayers, spent thousands of dollars caring for a lady who really didn't want medical care and who you couldn't help. Meanwhile, the young, relatively healthy woman nearly died because she couldn't buy insulin!"

Kate stood in silence as the reality sunk in. She shook her head and said, "It's horrible, but true."

"From the economic perspective, it seems pretty simple. Don't spend money on something that doesn't work. Instead, invest the resources you have in ways that create a benefit."

"It's not always that simple in medicine. We're talking about people's lives. It's complicated, Meg."

"I understand it's complicated, but it's obvious that she did not benefit and didn't want the care. She suffered needlessly, and all that money was wasted."

"You win." Kate smiled. "Let's finish our run. I'm hungry."

Meg smiled. "Let's just jog home, Speedy. I'm not done with my questions."

"I promise to jog." They both laughed and started up the path.

"That young woman should be able to get insulin," said Meg.

"Certainly."

"With our economy being so bad, I can't imagine more tax dollars being directed toward medical care. Can you?"

"I don't know where it will come from."

"There's an alternative, Kate. Use the resources more efficiently."

"Wisdom in government spending. Do those two go together?" Kate smiled.

Meg continued, "I just read that 64 percent of health care dollars are spent on about 10 percent of the population, and most of those patients are elderly."

"That fits with what I see at Mercy."

"I wonder how many elderly people end up in a situation like your patient. They wouldn't want that expensive medical care if they had the chance to decline it. I'm sure most people would reject it if they knew the trauma and futility of resuscitation attempts."

Meg continued, "If people knew how much was wasted on this futile end-of-life care, I think they'd ask their doctors to let them die naturally and not resuscitate."

"I agree. That's why Dr. Dawson keeps urging us to discuss Code status with patients."

"Tell me more about Dr. Dawson."

"He expects a lot from us. He demands that we work hard and treat our patients with respect. He also requires that we discuss Code status issues with our patients." She paused as her thoughts wandered. "He reminds me of Dad."

Meg smiled. "In what way?"

"You know how people felt at ease around Dad. His smile and voice were disarming, and people felt comfortable talking to him. Dr. Dawson's also committed to the residents and students like Dad was. You can tell he wants each of us to be a good doctor."

"I hope I can meet him."

"I'm sure you will, Meg. I'll ask him about these economic issues."

"Any other excitement?"

Kate rolled her eyes. "One of the senior residents is sort of a creep, and he's been coming on to me."

"What's going on?"

"He thinks he's quite the lady's man. He's always hitting on the interns and nurses. It's disgusting."

"There are jerks like him at the bank, too," Meg said.

"He dresses more like a banker than a resident. He thinks we should all bow down and worship him, even though he's only two years ahead of us. The worst part is, he's really smart."

"What's his name?"

"Jack Gerard. That is, *Doctor* Gerard." Kate smiled.

"Sounds like a cool guy." Meg smiled playfully.

"He was totally put off that I wouldn't go out with him for a drink after work two days ago. I don't think he's used to hearing 'No.'"

Meg laughed. "Doesn't sound like your type, Kate."

"He's definitely not. Anyway, I don't have time for romance right now. There'll be time for that later."

They jogged past Meg's apartment and said goodbye. Kate picked up the pace for the last half mile. She looked forward to quizzing Dr. Dawson on medical economics.

10

The next afternoon, Kate walked through the doors of the Mercy Medical Center Clinic for the first time. The commotion in the waiting room jolted her as two mothers fought to separate their brawling children. Kate stopped to keep an eye on the fight, thinking that it might turn nasty. Once the children were seated, the mothers' conflict escalated. Kate pulled out her cell phone, called security, and crossed the room, hoping to soothe the hostility.

Neither combatant noticed Kate's arrival. Their wild gestures and river of four-letter words made a scuffle increasingly likely. Kate watched the escalating frenzy. Then, hoping she could diffuse their anger, she shouted, "Ladies, could you please keep it down, you're scaring the children."

Both women stopped and glared at the tall, thin woman in a lab coat. Before they could say a word, Kate blurted, "I can get some candy for the kids to help them relax." Kate's pulse was racing as she tried to mask her fear.

The larger woman's glare softened. She smiled and said, "Maybe you can give a piece to this slimy little slut, too." Those words grabbed the attention of the packed waiting room.

Before the big woman knew what hit her, she collapsed under the blow of a metal chair across her brow. Blood flowed freely from a gaping laceration across her scalp. Kate jumped back, watching as the smaller woman kicked into the other woman's rib cage and then fell upon her, scratching at her face.

The fallen woman tried to ward off the attack. Kate screamed and pulled at the aggressor with little effect. Everyone in the packed waiting room stood to watch the ferocious beating. Finally the door burst open, and two security officers seized the wild attacker.

Kate reeled backward in disbelief. Several members of the clinic staff stood speechless. Conflict in the cramped waiting room was common, but it had been a long time since they'd seen all-out warfare.

A nurse emerged with gloved hands and a wad of gauze pads, which she pressed against the hemorrhaging wound to stem the flow. The woman was gradually awakening from the pounding and was able to answer simple questions. Kate and the clinic's attending physician, Dr. Jefferson, examined the patient and administered additional first aid. They transferred her to the ER with hopes they could resume their routine.

As Kate walked out of the waiting room, the nurse supervisor raised an eyebrow and said, "Welcome to the Mercy Clinic, Dr. Simon."

Kate snapped her bloodied gloves into the can and looked up. She was a little pale. She said, "Glad to be here…I guess."

Kate collected her thoughts as she sat in Dr. Jefferson's tiny windowless office in the middle of the clinic. Three other residents squeezed in, too. Charts formed three peaks across his desk. Once inside the office, he said, "We're already a half hour behind schedule, and we have about 40 patients to see this afternoon. You need to see the patients and discuss your findings and plans with me. I'll see them with you if I need to.

"Oh, and be sure to document everything carefully in the charts. We have so many different residents seeing patients, good records are essential. Never forget the medical-legal aspects of our records, too. If you don't document something, it never happened." He paused and then asked, "Any questions?"

The residents all sat silently, eager to get to work.

"Okay, let's get at it. Your first patients are in the exam rooms."

Each headed toward his or her respective patient. Kate's anticipation grew as she drew closer.

Kate removed the chart from the rack on the door and a broad smile broke over her face. As she opened the door, Toni Jackson met her with a big grin. Kate thrust her hand forward. "Good to see you, Toni. You look great," she said as she looked Toni over from head to toe. "How are you feeling?"

"I feel good. It's amazing what a little insulin can do." Toni's bright smile lifted Kate's spirits.

"What have your blood sugars been running?"

Toni looked down and the smile evaporated.

"What's up, Toni?"

"I have the glucose measuring machine, but I can't afford the test strips. Those things are expensive. I've tried to test my glucose a couple times, and today it was 133, which is good for me," said Toni.

Kate was frustrated and even angry—not at Toni, but at the system. All she could manage to say was, "That's really frustrating."

Kate bought some time to gain her composure by looking over the chart. She remembered Dr. Dawson telling her that nearly half of the public reports someone in their family skipping pills or postponing medical care they needed due to unaffordable costs.

Finally Kate asked, "Have you been more thirsty or hungry lately?"

"No, why's that?"

"When your blood sugar is high, you'll urinate more and be thirsty because you lose a lot of sugar in your urine. Watch out for that since you can't measure your blood sugar. You also need to watch for low blood sugars. Have you ever had low sugars?"

"Yeah, but not recently."

"So you know that if your sugar is low you will feel anxious and your heart rate will go up. You might feel hungry, too. Be sure to eat something sweet if you feel that way." Toni nodded and Kate continued, "Let me know if you have symptoms like that because we may need to adjust your insulin doses or your diet."

"Okay. I'll keep track of it."

Kate paused again, deep in thought. Finally she said, "Toni, I feel really bad that you can't afford to take care of yourself like you need to. Diabetes leads to all kinds of problems because it injures small blood vessels. It can lead to blindness, kidney failure, heart attacks, strokes, more infections, and neurological problems.

"If you control your blood sugar, all these complications are delayed—maybe for years. That's why I'd like you to monitor your glucose more regularly."

Toni shot right back, "I'd love to do that, and maybe someday I'll be able to. But for now, I can't. I need to get through college first, and then I can take better care of myself."

Kate looked down and said, "I know you'll do your best."

"There's one other thing, since we're talking money. Look at my hospital bill!" Toni pulled several pages out of her purse. She showed Kate the itemized list of hospital supplies and services.

Toni scanned down each column of charges and with her finger resting on the bottom bold number, said, "Three days, $13,543."

"What will you do?" asked Kate.

"The financial counselor from Mercy told me they adjusted my bill based on my income. I have to pay $4,000." Toni dropped her head and sighed. "That gives me another monthly payment on a broken budget. I don't know how I can do it."

Kate had never felt this helpless and outraged simultaneously. She wanted to scream. She sat in silence and finally said, "The clinic will be free, and I might be able to get you some test strips. We'll do the best we can."

Toni dropped her head again and after a long silence whispered, "I appreciate your concern, but I don't want charity." She looked back up at Kate and said, "I work really hard, and somehow I want to succeed."

"Why don't you let me help you? I really can't do much, but a little help could go a long way."

Toni didn't answer.

"Please think it over. Now, let's get to that exam."

Kate examined Toni efficiently and left the room to discuss her case with Dr. Jefferson. He returned with Kate to meet Toni. He reinforced the need for her to monitor her diet and insulin and put an exclamation point on the main point: "Don't stop your insulin!"

After he left, Kate wrote a prescription for insulin and provided a few additional instructions. She warned her that if she were to become nauseated and unable to keep food down, she should return to the clinic or hospital because of the danger of DKA.

Kate left Toni's room filled with apprehension and anger, knowing Toni's poverty would probably be a barricade to a healthy future.

Kate plopped down to write her note. After carefully documenting the visit per Dr. Jefferson's instructions, she pulled an index card covered with scribbles from her pocket. She gave it a speedy survey, crossed out one line, and then wrote, "Toni—test strips." Kate sat silently for a few seconds. Then she jumped up and high-tailed it to her next patient.

That afternoon passed in a flash. It was about five when she walked to the room of her final patient.

Outside the exam room, Kate rifled through Mrs. Maria Pelino's chart to review the basics: today's complaint, her medical problem list, and her medication list. Mrs. Pelino had been a patient in the clinic for several years but was new to Kate.

Mrs. Pelino stood, leaning in the corner reading a book, as Kate entered. Immediately Mrs. Pelino crossed the small room with her hand extended. "You must be Dr. Simon. I'm Maria Pelino. So nice to meet you," she said with a warm smile. Her dark Mediterranean features and Italian accent grabbed Kate's attention.

"I'm glad to meet you, Mrs. Pelino."

"Please call me Maria, if you don't mind, Doctor."

"Okay, Maria. I looked at your chart, and it says that you're 83 years old. Is that right?"

"Did you think I was older?" asked Maria with mock curiosity.

Kate chuckled and said, "Of course not. I thought you were about 65."

"I guess you know how to make friends, young lady."

Kate reviewed Mrs. Pelino's medical history and then began exploring Mrs. Pelino's life situation. She asked, "Do you live alone?"

"Yes. I like it that way."

"What do you mean?"

"I like to do things on my schedule and my way. After 83 years, I have the right to that, don't you think?" she said with an ornery grin.

"I won't take that away from you. Do you still drive?"

"Certainly. I have a 1986 Oldsmobile Cutlass that's in perfect shape. A young fella tried to buy it from me last week, but I'll never part with that beauty. It runs like a top."

Kate smiled in amazement and asked, "What do you do to keep busy?"

"I'm the director of the choir at the senior center and founder of the 'Knit-Wits.'"

Kate laughed and asked, "What in the world is that?"

Through a childish grin, she said, "That's our knitting and crocheting club. We're all a little crazy, so the name fits."

"It sounds like you're not sitting around home very much."

"Who wants to sit around when there are things to do?"

"I know you don't need much help, but do you have family or friends who can assist you?" asked Kate.

"I take care of my affairs, and I have a few young friends that can help me out. They're in their sixties." She smiled again.

"What about family? Do you have children, siblings, a husband?"

"I'm an only child. My husband has been dead for 10 years, and my son may as well be dead. I haven't seen him in years." Mrs. Pelino's face fell.

"What happened to your son?" asked Kate.

"He and I had a falling out after my husband's death. It was all over money, and we never worked it out." She glanced away and continued. "I miss Tommy, but I guess he's as stubborn as me, and so we live our own lives."

"That's sad, Mrs. Pelino. Have you tried to reach him lately?"

"No, I gave up a few years ago. He's getting on with his life. I have my friends here, so I'll just go about my life, too," she concluded.

"Maybe you should try again," suggested Kate.

"I'll think about it, but it's probably a lost cause."

"Okay, back to your other health issues. From what I can tell, everything is stable. Your blood pressure and cholesterol are under good control. If you keep those in check, you'll decrease the risk of heart attacks and strokes."

"I know. Dr. Hernandez, my last doctor here, always reminded me of that. He even convinced me to stop smoking two years ago."

"All right, let me examine you, and we'll wind things down."

Kate gave Mrs. Pelino a thorough exam and found a blowing sound in her neck: a bruit caused by turbulent blood flow across a plaque that narrows the artery. Normally there are no sounds over the carotid artery.

Kate asked, "Has anyone ever told you that you have a blowing sound in your neck?"

"Oh, yeah. Dr. Hernandez heard that about a year ago. He wanted to do some tests, but when he told me that it could lead to surgery, I said no."

Kate's tone turned grave and she asked, "Do you realize that this could signal a blockage in your artery that could cause a stroke?"

"That's what Dr. Hernandez told me. I'll tell you the same thing I told him. I don't want to have a bunch of tests and surgeries. I'm living a good life and don't want to get into all that. From what I hear, the surgery could even *cause* a stroke."

Kate slid forward in her chair and peered straight into Mrs. Pelino's eyes. "I guess you've made up your mind, but I want you to understand that you could have a stroke that could disable you or cause your death. We might be able to prevent that by looking into this. Are you sure you don't want to pursue it?"

"I'm certain. Thank you for asking though. I appreciate your concern."

"You're clearly of sound mind and have the right to refuse medical treatment." Then Kate flipped the chart open and pointed toward the medication list. She asked, "Are you taking aspirin?"

"I take a baby aspirin each day."

"Good. That could help prevent a stroke."

Kate looked down at the chart to determine whether anyone had discussed end-of-life issues with Mrs. Pelino. She leafed through several pages and saw nothing. Although she knew the importance of the discussion, she felt overwhelmed as she considered initiating it. She wished Dr. Dawson was there to take the lead.

She took a deep breath and asked, "Has anyone talked to you about end-of-life decisions?"

"What do you mean?"

"Has anyone ever discussed things like a Living Will, power of attorney, or Code status with you?" asked Kate, hoping that Dr. Hernandez or someone had already been into this issue with Mrs. Pelino.

"No, but I think I know what you're talking about. It's been a topic with the Knit-Wits lately."

"Why's that?"

"We've had a few friends die recently. One lady had a heart attack and suffered in the hospital for several weeks before she passed. We've been arguing over whether we would want to be treated that way."

Kate breathed a sigh of relief and said, "I'm glad you've discussed this. Lots of people avoid the topic until it's too late."

"Too late?"

"Right now you're healthy, your thinking is clear, and you can make decisions about your health care, but that could change. I want you to be able to specify what type of medical care you would want at the end of your life."

Mrs. Pelino waited for Kate to continue. "I foresee no imminent problems, but that bruit in your neck could cause problems, and at 83, you need to plan ahead."

"I want that, too."

"If you were in a situation where you needed your heart restarted or needed a breathing machine to keep you alive, would you want those measures?"

"No," she said and her head dropped. "I watched my husband and a few friends die. My husband had terrible lung disease. We liked our cigarettes. He was in and out of the hospital several times over his last two years of life. He was miserable. He ended up dying on a breathing machine in intensive care right across the street at Mercy."

Mrs. Pelino's tone was sober and resolute. "I don't want to go through that. I've lived a good life. I don't want to suffer like that. When my time comes, I'd like to die a natural death."

"That means that if your heart or breathing stops, you would not want to be revived?"

"That's absolutely right." She grasped Kate's hand with both of hers and said, "Young lady, you are the first doctor to talk to me like this. I could tell it wasn't easy for you, but I appreciate it."

Kate proceeded to relate the facts about resuscitation to Mrs. Pelino and encouraged her to convey those to her fellow Knit-Wits.

"Thank you! I'll talk to my friends. Many of them will want to discuss this with their doctors."

They exchanged farewells, and Kate asked her to schedule a follow-up visit in about two months. It was getting late as Kate sat down to finish the paperwork before she reviewed the case with Dr. Jefferson. The loud speaker cracked to life: *ping, ping, ping* and her adrenaline surged with the realization that she was on call. She jumped up and was sprinting for the door when she heard, *Code Blue Room 3048.*

Mrs. Pelino's chart lay incomplete on the desk. The staff filed it with the day's other paperwork; in the excitement of the Code, Kate forgot about it.

11

Kate walked into Mercy at 5:30 a.m. to start her second month of internship with a new team—a new senior resident and attending. Her attending was Dr. Harold Slone and senior resident, Dr. Jack Gerard. Kate hadn't worked with Jack since she'd rejected his advances and wondered how things would go.

As she got off the elevator, Kate watched Jack straighten his tie and push his hair back. He lifted his arm to reveal his Rolex.

Kate met a third-year med student, Jim Lowe, who would be part of their team for the month.

Jack strutted down the hall to meet Kate and Jim and said, "Let's get to work, kids. There's a lot to learn today, and we need to see a few patients before Dr. Slone gets here at eight."

Kate managed a smile and nodded to Jim. They picked up the charts and fell in line. Jack lifted his head high as he led his charges down the hall.

Their first patient was an elderly man admitted with congestive heart failure. Kate and Jim had reviewed the patient's history, and Kate updated Jack on his status and the plan of care.

While Kate spoke, Jack's eyes darted about. He pulled his BlackBerry out and began checking his messages. When Jack looked away, Kate glanced at Jim and rolled her eyes. When she finished talking, Jack asked, "What's your diagnosis, Dr. Simon?"

"Congestive heart failure."

"CHF is not a diagnosis," he said, looking up from his phone. "What's the *cause* of the CHF?" His eyes bore in on Jim.

Jim shifted from side to side and wrung his hands. He said, "I'm not sure, Dr. Gerard."

"You don't know?" He slipped his phone in its holster and took a step toward Jim. "Do you hope to be a doctor someday, son?"

"Yes sir," stammered Jim.

"Then you better learn what causes CHF, moron." Jim's head dropped and his shoulders slouched. Then Jack turned to Kate and demanded, "Give me five potential causes of CHF in this patient, Simon."

Kate took a deep breath. She'd been through this list before, but she was having trouble thinking with Jack bearing down on her. She hesitated for a few seconds, and before she could say a word,

Jack broke in. "You're a doctor, Simon, and you don't know a differential diagnosis for CHF? This is basic stuff, young lady."

Kate's frustration grew into anger, and her face flushed. She spit out her list in rapid fire succession: "Hypertension, myocardial infarction, kidney failure, cardiomyopathy, anemia."

Kate continued with mounting speed and intensity. "But the cause in this patient is poor compliance with his medical regimen. He stopped his meds two weeks ago and has been getting short of breath ever since." She took a deep breath and looked away in a vain effort to veil her increasing contempt. Kate could not comprehend this level of arrogance in a physician who was only two years her senior and still a resident.

Jim shook his head in disgust when he saw Jack's smile grow as he gloried in Kate's anger and frustration. Jack brushed back his dark hair and with calculated coolness said, "That's a pretty good list, Simon. Let's try to be more attentive in the future."

Jack leafed through the chart to review the plan of attack. Kate looked past Jack and took a few long, deliberate, slow breaths. Jack spun away and motioned toward the elevator. On the way, he grabbed his cell phone and rolled through the morning news as they waited for the elevator.

Next they approached the room of a 25-year-old woman, Ms. Janet Browning, who had been admitted for chest pain after using crack cocaine. Kate interviewed and examined her earlier that morning, and the memory of the conversation was etched vividly in Kate's mind.

She had asked Ms. Browning, "Do you know why crack causes chest pain?"

"I'm not sure, Doctor, but I know it happens a lot to me."

"Why did you come to the hospital this time?"

"The pain wouldn't go away."

"The cocaine causes constriction of blood vessels in your heart, and that decreases blood flow. The heart aches when it doesn't get the blood it needs. Besides, when you use cocaine, your heart beats faster and harder, so it needs more blood flow to give it oxygen." Kate hesitated and asked, "Do you understand, Ms. Browning?"

"Yes," she said as she dropped her head.

"Ms. Browning," Kate said and then stopped until the patient's eyes met hers. "Crack cocaine can cause a heart attack and kill you."

Her voice trembled. "I know. My sister died last week using crack and I'm scared. That's why I'm here. I want to get off this stuff."

Kate sighed, pulled a chair along the bed, and sat down. Janet's expression softened, and she kicked her legs over the side of the bed to sit up.

"How long have you been using?"

"I started when I was 15, so that makes about 10 years."

"How did you get started?"

"My mother and grandmother raised me. When I was 15, my mother was arrested, and we never saw her again. My grandmother was sick, so my sister and I ended up on the streets."

"Who did you live with?"

"We lived with our aunt for a while, but there wasn't room for us there. She had three kids of her own, and it was only a two-bedroom flat. My sister and I ended up on the streets."

"Then what?" Kate knew the answer.

"We met Johnny. He took care of us. He gave us a place to stay and food, and then he put us to work."

"What did you do?" Kate winced inside with the question.

"We did whatever we needed to do to make money."

The answer seemed obvious by now. She'd heard stories like this before. Kate tried to make it easier for Janet to tell the truth. Kate asked, "Did you live as a prostitute?"

Janet's head dropped again, and she whispered, "Yeah. We didn't have much choice. He took good care of us, and there was always plenty of crack."

Kate waited for Janet to look up again and asked, "Do you really want to get off the crack?"

"Yeah."

"It'll be tough. You'll have to quit the crack and change your whole way of life. Are you ready to do that?"

"I want to try. I'm only 25 and I don't want to die."

Kate grabbed her hand. "Listen Janet, I'll do everything I can to get you into rehab and help you out, but it's going to take a big commitment from you."

"I have a cousin who went through rehab, and the people at her church helped her through it. She told me I could come live with her, if I go through rehab."

"That's great, Janet. Most people don't have that kind of help. I'll get our social worker to come by and see if we can get you into one of the area programs."

Kate would never forget the expression of gratitude on Janet's face as she left the room and now was looking forward to seeing her again with the team.

When they arrived outside Janet's door, Jack put his BlackBerry away and asked, "What's her story?"

Kate summarized the history and physical, and concluded, "She had chest pain from crack cocaine use and is interested in drug rehabilitation."

Jack shook his head and asked, "What did her EKG and cardiac enzymes show?"

"They were normal."

"No heart attack. Get that crack whore out of here."

Kate took a step back like she'd been slugged in the gut. Then she faced Jack squarely. "Would you repeat that, *Doctor* Gerard?"

Jack put the chart down and took a step toward Kate. "I said, get the *crack whore* out of here."

Kate knew this was about to get ugly, and the risks of being on Jack's bad side swirled through her head. She couldn't accept his cruelty.

"Are you saying that we shouldn't try to treat her addiction? She told me that she wanted help."

"C'mon, Simon. You can't believe her. She's probably just looking for a soft bed and a few warm meals for another day."

"So you're convinced she's hopeless?"

"That's right."

"How many of our other patients do you think are hopeless?" Kate's intensity swelled.

Jack looked around the hall and moved even closer to Kate. She stood her ground. He gritted his teeth and sneered. "After you've seen how many of these addicts milk the system and never change, you'll wake up."

"You're wrong."

Kate could see Jack's fury building. She could tell he was not used to being confronted.

Jack leaned even closer. "I'm in charge of this service, and I order you to discharge this patient. Today. Do you understand?"

Kate crossed her arms and stepped back. "Are you forbidding me from getting her help with her addiction?"

Jack stared long and hard into Kate's unblinking eyes. She knew the request was reasonable.

Finally Jack blurted, "Look, I don't care what you do as long as she's discharged today. I don't want to see her again." With that, Jack turned and walked away.

Kate and Jim stood in silence, watching Dr. Gerard's swaggering exit. Jim looked at Kate and asked, "Are you sure you want to get into a war with Gerard?"

"I didn't have much choice, did I?"

"You always have a choice, and you chose to start a war. He won't forget this."

"Some things are worth fighting about."

"You better be careful. He could take you down, and he seems like the kind of person who might enjoy ruining someone's career."

"He's a lot of talk. I'll treat people with respect, and he can do what he wants." Kate glanced at her watch and said, "We better get going. We need to meet up with Dr. Slone in 15 minutes. You call the psychiatrist, and I'll contact the social worker. Tell the psychiatrist that we need to get her discharged today."

They accomplished their mission of mercy and met Dr. Dawson on the way to the ICU.

"Hi Kate. Did you see that young woman we took care of a few weeks ago with DKA?"

"Yes, Toni Jackson."

"How's she doing?"

"Real well. That reminds me. I have some questions about medical costs. Would you have time to talk after conference today?"

"Sure. Let's meet up about one o'clock."

"See you then."

12

After the lunchtime conference, Kate met up with Dr. Dawson.

"Toni Jackson brought her bill with her to the clinic, and it blew my mind."

"Medical care is a little pricier than you imagined?"

"Not just a little! That cost about $14 grand!"

"I remember she was quite concerned about the bill. Did they work out a payment plan for her?"

Kate grimaced and sarcastically said, "They knocked it all the way down to $4,000." She continued, "Toni's anxious about paying her bills and simply surviving. I'm worried she won't take care of herself because of the cost. She can't even afford to check her blood sugar."

"Doesn't seem right, does it?" Dr. Dawson muttered.

"My sister and I talked about these ethical and financial issues we face every day.

"Remember, Toni developed DKA because she couldn't afford a $40 vial of insulin. Then we resuscitated the elderly woman and put her in the ICU until her daughter decided to withdraw care. My sister asked me, 'How much did it cost to resuscitate that lady and keep her alive?' I don't have a clue. Can you tell me?"

Dr. Dawson took a deep breath and sighed. "What did it cost to care for that lady? It's not easy or simple to answer that one. I know it should be, but here's the rub. Did they teach you about DRGs in med school?"

"I don't remember," she said and then paused. "Maybe the 'G' is some type of goiter?" They both laughed.

"Not a goiter. Diagnosis Related Group, and it means everything to hospitals and Medicare. It's too bad they don't teach this stuff in most medical schools, but here's the short course.

"Medicare is our national health insurance for people over the age of 65 who have paid into the system, and for permanently disabled people. When a Medicare patient comes into the hospital, the hospital gets paid based on the diagnosis—the ailment that caused admission.

"If a patient has pneumonia, then the hospital gets a set fee based on the diagnosis. It's a good system in many ways, because it forces the hospital and doctors to be as cost-effective as possible to increase the profit margin for the hospital."

"So you're saying that the hospital gets a set fee for taking care of Medicare patients based solely on the diagnosis?"

Dr. Dawson replied, "In general, that's the case. It's complicated by modifiers in the case of unanticipated problems and additional diagnoses, but if we stick to the big picture, that's it." He continued, "So the cost to Medicare, or the taxpayer, if you want to look at it that way, would be the DRG."

"That's exactly what I want to know, Dr. Dawson," said Kate as her pace quickened. "My sister, Meg, asked me all about the economics, and I didn't have any good answers for her. I want to know how much that resuscitation cost the medical system. In retrospect, it was unwanted, unnecessary, unfruitful, and caused her needless pain. It consumed financial resources that could be used for people like Toni."

Kate continued, "Can we find out the cost of the DRG for Mrs. Frank?"

Dr. Dawson looked at his watch and said, "Come on. I've got 15 minutes, and we can go talk to Dr. Jim Zwick in administration. He'll be able to help us."

They hurried down the hall and took the elevator to the twelfth floor. A receptionist met them and called Dr. Zwick. He hobbled out of his office on crutches and with a brace on his left leg.

"What happened to you, Jim?"

"I wrecked my bike last week on wet pavement and injured my knee, but I'm fine. The bike didn't fare as well." They both laughed.

"We wondered if you had time for a few questions," Dr. Dawson said. He turned toward Kate. "This is Kate Simon, one of our interns. We've been talking about health care costs, and we wondered if you could help us out."

"I'll do what I can. You know part of my job is trying to keep us out of the red here at Mercy. It's not an easy job," he chuckled. "Come into the conference room."

Kate knew they didn't have much time, so she got right to the point. "Dr. Zwick, I'm trying to figure out how all this works. They didn't teach us much about it in medical school," she said with a smile. "Dr. Dawson told me about DRGs, and we were wondering if you could give us some real numbers."

"I probably can. What diagnosis were you looking at?" he asked.

"We had a recent case of a lady who had Sick Sinus Syndrome that caused her to pass out. After she was admitted, she coded on the floor, went to the ICU, and died there when we changed her Code status to Comfort Care. We'd like to know what that cost."

Dr. Zwick answered, "I don't have that on the top of my head, but give me a few seconds and I can pull that up on my laptop."

Dr. Zwick pecked away at his keyboard for about a minute. "The payment for Sick Sinus Syndrome complicated with a heart attack is $4,261."

Dr. Dawson and Kate looked at each other in disbelief. Even Dr. Dawson had gotten out of touch with how much medical care cost. Then Kate asked, "So that's how much Medicare pays Mercy for the care we provided to the patient?"

"That's right." Dr. Zwick paused and then continued, "The real cost is another matter. We could figure that all out, but for your purposes, the DRG cost is the best thing to go with."

"What you're saying is, the taxpayers paid $4,261 to cover this DRG."

"You've got it."

Kate sat silently for a few moments and then asked, "Do you have time for a few more quick questions?"

"Sure," responded Dr. Zwick.

"Do you think the government is going to commit more taxpayer money to health care to cover these costs as people are getting older?"

"It's not really up to the government. It's up to us taxpayers, and I think most people feel like we spend too much on health care now. Here's the problem. Our population is aging, and costs will continue to escalate, but people don't want to spend more on health care."

Kate thought this through and then said, "Here's how I see it. Tell me if you think I'm crazy." She stood up and went to the whiteboard. "Do you mind if I write these points out? It helps me clarify my thoughts."

Dr. Dawson and Dr. Zwick looked at each other with amusement, and Dr. Dawson said, "Go right ahead."

Kate turned to the board and wrote, "LIMITED RESOURCES." Then she said, "We have limited resources since we spend a lot on health care and taxpayers don't want to spend more." She looked at the two physicians, who nodded in agreement.

Next she wrote, "AGING POPULATION," and said, "You just said that expenditures are going up since the population is aging."

Again both nodded in agreement.

Next she wrote, "UNWANTED/UNNECESSARY CARE," and said, "In the case we just discussed, the expenditure of $4,261 was totally unnecessary. If someone would have discussed Code status with her daughter months ago, we could have allowed her to die naturally without prolonging her death."

"Neither one of us will argue that point, Dr. Simon," said Dr. Dawson.

Finally she wrote, "TONI JACKSON." Dr. Zwick raised an eyebrow, and Dr. Dawson straightened in his seat, wondering where his intern was headed.

Kate took a deep breath and began, "Toni Jackson, Dr. Zwick, is a 22-year-old single woman who was on our service last month. We admitted her for DKA. The cause of her DKA was non-compliance. She didn't take her insulin because she couldn't afford it!" She paused and thought for a few seconds.

She turned to the board and pointed to the first line, LIMITED RESOURCES. "We all agree that there are limited resources. No one is ready to write a blank check for medical care, right?" She looked at her two superiors, and they nodded in agreement.

She pointed to the line UNWANTED/UNNECESSARY CARE. Her tone and pace elevated. She said, "Why can't we stop spending our limited resources on unwanted and unnecessary care so that we can spend them *here?*" Then she stabbed her finger toward TONI JACKSON.

Dr. Dawson looked down at his watch and jumped up. "You've put your finger on an issue that has many people bewildered. We'll have to work on it later because you and I need to get going."

13

Kate paged Jack and hurried to meet the team on the general medical unit. She wondered what torture Jack would inflict this afternoon. As she arrived on the floor, he glanced up and wondered aloud, "So why is our young Dr. DoGood so late?"

Kate rolled her eyes.

Jack went on. "I like that name. 'Dr. DoGood.' Has a nice ring to it."

Kate was not in the mood for more insults and simply replied, "I lost track of time. Sorry I'm late."

"Let's not get into any bad habits. I'd hate to see you lose your job. All your drug addicts and prostitutes would miss you if you end up on the street yourself," Jack said with a wicked smirk.

The abuse ended when Jack's annoying cell phone rang with Robert Palmer's *Bad Case of Loving You (Doctor, Doctor)*. He let the tune play a few bars before answering the call. Jack listened intently, ended the call and turned to Kate.

"All right, DoGood, I have another case for you in the ER. There's a little chick down there in DKA. Her landlord called the cops to open her apartment when he hadn't seen her for a few days. She's almost dead. Go see what you can do and call me."

DKA—the same condition Kate had warned Toni about in the clinic. Her head spun as she considered the possibility. Without a word, she turned and sprinted at Code speed to the ER.

14

Kate walked into Room 54 and confirmed her worst fear—Toni Jackson. What could have happened? Kate had thoroughly discussed DKA with Toni and urged her to get to the hospital if she developed threatening symptoms. Kate was overwhelmed to see Toni on the ventilator with all the requisite tubes. She touched her and recoiled. Toni was cool as a corpse.

Kate discussed the situation with the ER attending physician, Dr. Bowman, and found that Toni had a urinary tract infection that had apparently triggered her DKA. She was probably taking her insulin, but the infection precipitated the DKA.

Kate was not thinking clearly, but the attending reminded her that during Toni's recent hospitalization she had a urinary catheter, which probably caused the infection. He also reminded her that diabetics are prone to UTIs.

He also told her that Toni was doing terribly. He said, "It looks like this young lady was down for a long time—maybe a day or more before they found her. Her blood pressure's bottoming out, and her heart's racing."

He saw the emotion in Kate's eyes and asked, "Do you know this patient?"

Kate's voice trembled. "Yeah, she's my patient. Is there anything else we can do?"

"I'm doing everything possible, and she's still headed south," said Dr. Bowman. "She's gotten four liters of fluid, and I'm giving her more as fast as I can. She's on IV pressors, too, and her blood pressure is still low. She's also on IV insulin, and we gave her antibiotics."

Kate knew she needed to act quickly to help Dr. Bowman, but so many questions were swirling through her mind. She wondered why Toni didn't call or come to the ER. And then the realization hit her—*the bill.*

Toni couldn't handle the first bill. The thought of a second one must have paralyzed her.

After examining Toni and conferring with Dr. Bowman, Kate decided there was nothing else they could do but continue the present therapies and wait. She sat helplessly at Toni's bedside, thinking of what she must have gone through in that lonely apartment. She probably had burning with urination. The next day, a fever would have developed. She would have started to feel nauseated as the DKA rolled along. Then increasing shortness of breath, confusion, and finally she would have slipped into a stupor. Kate's jaw clenched as she imagined the scene.

Since she'd been in the ER, her condition continued to deteriorate. Jack and Dr. Slone joined Kate in the ER. They all did their best to revive Toni, but nothing helped. DKA won; Toni lost. When her heart stopped, resuscitation was futile. Plenty of care and cost, but too late to make a difference.

A wonderful young woman lost to poverty and pride.

Kate finished her day in a trance and looked forward to meeting Meg for coffee.

15

Meg was sitting outside, sipping a latté, enjoying a late summer evening when Kate peddled up. Kate methodically chained her bike and walked in the door without looking for Meg. After getting her drink, Kate made it through the door, where Meg caught sight of her red, swollen eyes. She stood up to reach over and hug her sister. "Kate, what happened?"

"I lost my first patient today. Remember that young college student I told you about? The one that needed the $40 vial of insulin and worried about her hospital bill? She died."

"She died?" Meg gasped.

Kate dropped her head, and they both sat down. "She got a urinary tract infection and developed DKA again. We did everything, but it was too late. She was essentially dead before she got to the hospital."

"Why didn't she go to the hospital sooner?"

"I'm not sure." Kate paused. "But I think I know, and that's what's driving me crazy." Kate stopped again.

"You think it was the bill?"

Kate sighed and wiped her eyes. "I'm sure it was. I can't get the vision of her out of my head. Sitting alone, hoping the symptoms would improve, and hoping she wouldn't have to go to the hospital."

Meg grabbed Kate's hand and said, "This is so unfair. How could this happen in this city? In this country?"

They sat silently for a few minutes. Now they knew the truth. There were health care dollars to spend, but people like Toni were cut out of a system that spends millions on unwanted and unnecessary care...while people like Toni die.

Meg finally blurted out, "Our health care system is pitiful!"

Kate paused, considering Meg's outburst, and countered, "Yeah, there are some really bad things about our system, but some parts are really good."

"What's good about it?"

"We are the best in the world at saving people. Remember that young father with the heart attack I told you about? The American health care system is the best in the world for urgent problems.

"Our system is good at saving lives, but we end up prolonging lives in people that have no hope. Then we don't have resources to care for poor people like Toni." Kate's eyes were clearing.

Meg interjected, "I've done some more study about that since our last talk. You won't believe this. I found that 30 percent of Medicare dollars are spent on the last year of life even though only five percent of Medicare patients die yearly." She reached into her purse, pulled out a memo, and read, "The mean annual Medicare expenditures for the last 12 months of life in the elderly rose from $1,924 in 1976 to about $23,000 in 1995."

"That's mind blowing on one hand but fits with what I see at Mercy," said Kate.

"I wonder what people in America would do if they understood this fact?" asked Meg.

They discussed that question for a long time, and both left the coffee shop resolved to do what they could to fight for people like Toni Jackson.

16

A week later on September 1, Kate rolled into the parking lot at about 5:30 a.m. to start her third month at Mercy. With the new month came a new list of patients and a change in her team. She was glad to be back on service with Dr. Dawson, but she would still have to contend with Dr. Gerard, whose image caused a fleeting wave of nausea.

She saw her patients efficiently and found them to be in good condition. She had learned so much in only two months. That was one good thing to be said for long hours.

Despite the problems, she was glad to be a physician. As she considered the terrible tragedy of Toni Jackson, she was not cynical or defeated. Instead, she had a growing sense that these financial issues and inequities could be overcome.

The team met in the ICU to review the two new admissions. Dr. Gerard met her with his typical greeting. "Good morning, Dr. DoGood," he said with disdain. Kate still found it difficult to imagine why this man was a physician. Jack was always careful to conceal his nastiness toward Kate from Dr. Dawson.

Dr. Neil Patel was her fellow intern for the month. Neil was a graduate of Penn State and grew up in eastern Ohio; his family emigrated from India when he was a child. Like Kate, Neil looked forward to a career in Family Medicine. Kate and Neil shared intern duties, and this was his first month with Dr. Gerard. Neil had been on call the previous night, so he had the job of presenting the new patients to the team. Kate was glad that Dr. Dawson would be their attending physician for the month.

Dr. Dawson pointed the way toward their first patient, and Dr. Patel began. "The next case is an elderly lady who presented with a chief complaint of being unable to talk and move her right side." He continued, "This is an 83-year-old woman who is a patient in our clinic with a history of hypertension and a carotid bruit."

Kate's pulse raced as she thought of her patient Mrs. Pelino.

Dr. Patel continued as they stood near the door. "The patient was having lunch with a friend when she suddenly developed weakness and couldn't speak."

Kate broke from the team and grabbed the chart. The stroke victim was Mrs. Pelino.

Kate's thoughts raced. "I wish she would have listened to me about that carotid bruit. That was probably the cause of this." As she thought more about Mrs. Pelino, she remembered her clearly stated wishes about her medical care: no testing, no special procedures, no surgeries. She remembered Mrs. Pelino saying she would rather live a good life than a long one. She'd lived 83 good years and was happy with that.

Kate returned to the team, and Dr. Patel was discussing Mrs. Pelino's history. "Apparently Mrs. Pelino was at the clinic a few weeks ago, but there is no note on the chart. I'm not sure who saw her, and I don't know what they did."

Kate's mouth went dry, and her heart was pounding. Not only was Mrs. Pelino in bad shape, but Kate recognized that she had really screwed up. She pushed forward and said, "I made a big mistake. I saw this patient in the clinic. They called a Code while I was finishing up. I rushed off and forgot to finish the chart."

Kate saw Jack try to suppress a smile as he watched her squirm.

Dr. Dawson spoke up. "That is a big mistake. You remember what I've told you, 'If you don't document it, it didn't happen.' You can't let this happen. It's a critical mistake." His voice was stern, and his eyes locked with Kate's.

She nodded and glanced away, but said nothing. The team stood silently. Jack watched Kate's every move from the corner of his eye, relishing her calamity.

Dr. Dawson broke the silence. "Do you remember what you did?"

"Yes. I did a full history and physical since it was our first visit. I found a carotid bruit and saw that her previous physician had addressed it with her. I gave her the options, including evaluation of the bruit, but she did not want to pursue testing."

"Anything else?" asked Dr. Dawson.

"I discussed Code status with her. She told me that she would not want to be coded and she would not accept any type of artificial life support." Kate's stomach felt like it was tied in knots.

"Hopefully she'll be alert enough to reaffirm that decision. If not, we can talk things over with her family," said Dr. Dawson.

Kate's heart sank. "That could be a problem. She had a falling out with her only son after her husband's death, and they haven't spoken for years."

"That might complicate things," said Dr. Dawson, shaking his head. He shrugged, turned toward the room, and then continued, "Let's see her now, and we'll figure that out later."

Dr. Dawson examined Mrs. Pelino. She was very sleepy and couldn't speak. She moved her left side but not her right side. Her eyes moved, and at times she made eye contact.

Dr. Dawson explained that these were signs of a large stroke on the left side in the middle part of the brain: a cerebral vascular accident.

After examining her, Dr. Dawson said, "Her prognosis is very poor. With a stroke this size, she could get a lot worse before she gets better."

"Why's that?" Neil asked.

"A large portion of the brain has been deprived of oxygen and that damaged tissue will become swollen. Since the skull is rigid, the edematous brain will push against the healthy brain and cause further damage. We will need to watch her electrolytes and blood pressure very closely. The neurology service has already been consulted, right?"

"Yes, sir."

Dr. Dawson turned to Kate. "Contact her son ASAP about her Code status since she can't communicate. I doubt that she'll improve substantially. That means end-of-life decisions will fall to her son."

"I'll get in touch with him," said Kate as she left Dr. Dawson. Kate turned to the med student and said, "We wouldn't be in this mess if I'd documented that conversation. I hope I can clean it up with her son."

17

Early that afternoon Kate's cell phone rang. It was the ICU nurse, and she was hopeful. "We contacted Mrs. Pelino's son, and he's on his way from about two hours away. He said he hasn't seen his mom for 10 years."

The nurse paused and Kate asked, "Anything else?"

"Yeah, he was really upset and said something like 'I won't let her down again.'"

"What do you think he meant?"

"I'm not sure."

"What's his name and number? I need to call him about Code status," said Kate.

The nurse rattled off the number and said goodbye.

Kate immediately called and Mr. Pelino answered. She was a bundle of nerves as she began, "Mr. Pelino, this is Dr. Kate Simon. I'm one of the doctors helping care for your mother. I want to update you and ask you a few questions."

"Sure. Go ahead. I appreciate the call."

"Your mother has had a very large stroke. She is awake but unable to communicate, and she can't move her right side."

"Oh, no! I was hoping to talk to her." He sounded like a man begging for his own life.

"I'm sorry, Mr. Pelino. She could improve, but I want you to know that it's likely her condition will decline due to swelling in the brain that occurs with a sizable stroke."

"Do you think she is going to die?" he gasped.

"Well, I'm afraid that's possible." Kate paused and continued, "There's something else I need to talk to you about. Your mother told me—" Mr. Pelino cut her off in midstream.

"Do your best to save her. I can't lose her."

Kate was not sure how to proceed, and she wished that Dr. Dawson was part of this difficult conversation.

"I spoke with your mother in the clinic recently. She told me she would not want to be kept alive if it required heroic measures. She told me that she would rather let nature take its course as long as she was kept comfortable."

His voice thundered, "Listen, Doctor, my mom would never say anything like that. I know she would want to live as long as she could. I want you to do everything to keep her alive." He paused and Kate was silent. Then he growled, "Do you understand? *Everything!*"

This was going from bad to worse. "We are doing everything, and we will continue to. When you arrive, my supervisor Dr. Dawson and I will talk to you."

He said, "I'll be there in 90 minutes," and hung up.

Kate called Dr. Dawson. "I just spoke with Mrs. Pelino's son. I filled him in on the stroke, but when we talked about Code status he got angry. He told me to do everything. Obviously, he's not ready to consider her desires."

"Since he's next of kin, we'll honor his wishes. We don't have your conversation documented or witnessed, so that carries little weight if he decides against it. I'm sure he's very upset. We'll talk to him when he arrives and help him understand the situation. Maybe he'll come around."

"I feel horrible about this. She was so clear about her wishes. Is there anything else I can do?"

"Not now. Just call me when Mr. Pelino arrives." His manner was abrupt, and Kate sensed his frustration at being thrust into this dilemma.

Kate went about her other duties but had a hard time shaking the feelings of shame and anxiety for Mrs. Pelino. She hoped Mrs. Pelino's son would have a change of heart, but that prognosis looked about the same as Mrs. Pelino's—grim.

18

Kate felt much more secure as she headed toward the ICU with Dr. Dawson leading. He'd been through difficult circumstances before, and Kate knew he would act in Mrs. Pelino's best interest. She also knew that he believed her about her conversation with Mrs. Pelino.

When they entered the room, Mr. Pelino was standing at the bedside. He was tall, tan, and fit, and appeared younger than his 62 years. He looked apprehensive and shifted back and forth as they approached.

Dr. Dawson offered a handshake and said, "I'm Dr. Dawson. Are you Thomas Pelino?" Mr. Pelino nodded, offering his hand.

"I'm one of your mother's doctors. This is Dr. Simon, who talked to you on the phone. Dr. Simon is one of our interns who saw your mother in the clinic recently."

"That's what she told me." He refused to look at Kate. "Please tell me how Mother is doing."

Dr. Dawson described the situation much like Kate had on the phone. Mr. Pelino was an intelligent man and asked good questions. He seemed to understand the severity of the illness and the prognosis.

Dr. Dawson told him that his mother could die from the stroke or from common complications such as pneumonia, blood clots, infections, and extension or worsening of the stroke.

After explaining the disease and treatments, Dr. Dawson moved to the Code status issue. "Dr. Simon told me that you and she discussed your mother's wishes regarding end-of-life decisions. You know, your mother told Dr. Simon that she would not want her life prolonged by artificial means."

Mr. Pelino erupted, "I heard what she said, and I don't believe her."

Dr. Dawson remained calm and said, "I have no reason not to believe her."

"I don't believe her, and I will not discuss this. I want you to do everything for my mom. I can't lose her. I lost her for the last 10 years, and I can't lose her now," he said, as his voice trailed off.

"Would you mind telling me about the last 10 years?" Dr. Dawson asked with genuine kindness and concern.

"After Dad died, Mom and I had a big argument about the estate. There was a life insurance policy that I thought was mine," he whispered.

"What happened?"

"Mom and I are stubborn and never reconciled. She tried. She wrote me a few letters. I never replied. It's my fault." He paused, looked Dr. Dawson straight in the eyes, and said, "I want you to get her better so I can talk to her again."

"Mr. Pelino, I'm sorry but I think it's unlikely that she will improve. I want to be honest with you. It's more likely that she'll get worse. We'll do what we can."

"I appreciate that, Doctor," said Mr. Pelino, as he turned back toward his mother.

Dr. Dawson turned to leave the room. Then slowly, almost reluctantly, he turned back toward Mr. Pelino. "Please think about the end-of-life questions. We're in a difficult situation.

"We believe your mother does not want heroic measures to keep her alive, and it is very likely she will need those. Since you are the next of kin, we are going to follow your wishes. We'll do everything we can to sustain her life."

Mr. Pelino did not look away from his mother and said, "I expect you to do *everything*."

They walked silently until they were outside the ICU. Then Kate erupted, "I can't believe this guy, and I can't believe I've screwed this up so badly. I'm sorry, Dr. Dawson. Now you're caught in the middle of this mess."

"You definitely screwed up, Kate, but his error is worse. He's obviously full of guilt about their relationship, and he's probably been bitter for a long time. He wanted to patch things up but never did. And here we are."

Dr. Dawson continued, "He wants to be her hero and believes he's helping her when, in fact, he's acting directly against her wishes."

"Guilt is powerful," Kate said.

"Sure is. But this is just the first day. Mr. Pelino is a sharp guy, and we need to give him some time. Just take good care of Mrs. Pelino, and I'll see you tomorrow morning," he said, as they parted ways.

The next week was not a good one for Mrs. Pelino or for Kate.

19

A first-year medical student accompanied Kate two days later on rounds, and Kate took her along to see Mrs. Pelino. Kate demonstrated the right-sided weakness and Mrs. Pelino's inability to speak or write messages. Finally she said to the student, "We need to check her gag reflex."

Kate informed Mrs. Pelino, "I'm going to press this wooden tongue depressor against the back of your throat. It might make you gag or cough." Mrs. Pelino did not make eye contact or acknowledge any understanding of Kate's warning. When Kate pressed the tongue depressor into her throat, Mrs. Pelino coughed ever so softly.

Kate turned to the student. "That's very weak." Kate continued, "Our gag reflex protects our airway from solids or fluids passing into the lungs. Stroke patients with a weak gag can't protect their airway and are at risk of aspiration pneumonia."

The med student gave a blank look, so Kate explained, "Aspiration pneumonia is an infection of the lung caused by material passing into the airways and lungs."

Kate continued, "We'll keep her head elevated about 30 degrees to help prevent aspiration, watch for a fever, and examine her regularly for signs of pneumonia."

Two days later, Mrs. Pelino developed aspiration pneumonia, despite their efforts to prevent it. The first sign was fever. The chest X-ray confirmed pneumonia.

Dr. Dawson explained the situation to the team and Thomas Pelino, who sat on the opposite side of the bed. "Your mother has pneumonia. It's caused because she is weak and unable to protect her airway. Remember, I told you a few days ago this was possible since her gag reflex is weak."

"I remember. How will you treat it?"

"With antibiotics through the IV."

"How soon will it resolve?"

"It could take several days. The primary adversary your mom faces is the weakness caused by the stroke. She can't generate a strong cough to clear infected fluids from her lungs. Coughing also opens her lungs back up." Dr. Dawson followed the shallow movements of her chest and continued, "Unfortunately, she may get worse."

Mr. Pelino stood, leaned across the bed, and asked, "What will you do if she gets worse?"

"She may deteriorate and be unable to breathe on her own. At that point, we would have to decide whether or not to put her on a breathing machine," Dr. Dawson said.

Mr. Pelino leaned even closer toward Dr. Dawson and snapped, "What do you mean, 'Whether or not to put her on a breathing machine'? I told you I want everything done. If Mom needs a machine, then start one. You better not let her die of pneumonia."

"I understand your wishes, but if her condition changes, we need to continue to talk. Since her condition is declining, I wanted to know if you had changed your mind."

"My decisions have been clear, and I would appreciate it if you and your staff would stop harassing me," he said through gritted teeth.

"I understand your wishes, Mr. Pelino, and we will continue Full Code care. I want to warn you that it is very likely, if not certain, that your mother will end up needing a ventilator. We would have to further sedate her and place a breathing tube into her airway to use the ventilator."

Dr. Dawson paused a few seconds and said, "The other issue is nutrition. We're feeding your mother through the tube in her nose that goes into her stomach, but we will need a permanent solution. Do you want us to proceed with the permanent feeding tube? We call that a gastric tube or G tube."

"Of course," he fired back.

"We'll have a surgeon stop by to discuss the G tube," Dr. Dawson added as he led the team out of the room. This was their last stop, so he left the team and headed toward his office.

Kate spent her free time at Mrs. Pelino's bedside, trying to comfort her. She spoke to her softly. "Maria, I'm so sorry. I've let you down. I know you didn't want to die like this. I'll do everything I can to help you."

Kate adjusted the feeding tube in her nostril to relieve pressure. She watched carefully for accumulation of saliva in her mouth and suctioned the fluids frequently.

Kate wondered how much pain Mrs. Pelino might be experiencing. Kate thought of the stiffness and pain that her own young, fit body sometimes felt from sleeping in an awkward position, and realized that Mrs. Pelino had been on her back and sides for days.

Kate was glad they could use analgesics to relieve all the pain Mrs. Pelino must be experiencing.

One day while in the room with Jack, Kate noticed swelling in Mrs. Pelino's hand around an IV site. The IV fluid had infiltrated into the surrounding tissue, a common and benign complication, but painful. "More unwanted agony," said Kate as she sniffled.

"So Dr. DoGood, this case of yours is a great one. A stroked-out old woman who can't die in peace because of a bitter son. Or should I say because her doctor didn't take good notes? What are you going to do?" he asked.

Kate stared Jack straight in the eye for several seconds, collecting her thoughts. "I'm going to do something that you know nothing about." She paused again, now glaring at Jack. He finally looked away and Kate said, "I'm going to treat her with care and dignity because I'm her doctor." Kate turned and left Jack standing in silence. If not before, Jack was her enemy now.

Things went as Dr. Dawson predicted. Mrs. Pelino's aspiration pneumonia got the best of her, and she required a ventilator to maintain adequate oxygen levels. The surgeon placed the G tube. Her heart and kidneys remained strong through the whole ordeal. She maintained a normal heart rhythm, good blood pressure, and good urine flow. Her fever and pneumonia gradually resolved.

What didn't improve was her weakness. It looked like the effects of the stroke would be permanent. She had no movement in her right side, and she became weaker and weaker on the other side due to lack of activity. Mrs. Pelino was dying, but her son would not let her go.

Kate suffered every day watching Mrs. Pelino suffer, knowing she could have prevented this agony with a few lines of documentation. Kate agonized, too, knowing the enormous expense of this unwanted health care. She wondered how many people like Toni Jackson could thrive, if the system did not spend endlessly on unnecessary care like this.

Kate was pretty certain Mrs. Pelino would not last long and believed that she would soon be at peace. But Kate underestimated Mrs. Pelino's strength, and she also underestimated her own impending dilemma.

20

Mrs. Pelino's growing weakness made it impossible to wean her from the ventilator. They tried four times to decrease the support of the ventilator and let her breathe independently, but each time she became short of breath and her oxygen levels dropped. Each time Kate watched in agony as Mrs. Pelino struggled for every breath, feeling Mrs. Pelino's pain as her own.

The doctors finally concluded that Mrs. Pelino needed to remain on the ventilator for the rest of her life, however long that agony might last. Therefore, she would need the surgeon to perform a tracheostomy, creating a hole in her trachea for a permanent breathing tube.

Thomas Pelino decided to proceed with surgery. Kate could only think how much Mrs. Pelino must detest this torture. Why couldn't he just let her go and not prolong her dying? And now, more unnecessary expenses. Kate felt sick, knowing this was all her fault.

The tracheostomy procedure was uneventful, and Mrs. Pelino remained stable. "The curse of a strong heart," thought Kate. She had weathered the storm of pneumonia and now lingered in this semi-vegetative state. Periodically she awakened enough to feel breathlessness and pain, yet she was not strong enough to improve.

While making rounds, Kate asked Dr. Dawson, "How long do you think Mrs. Pelino will live?"

He thought for a few seconds and said, "She's surprised me already. I'm amazed that she recovered from aspiration pneumonia and survived the ICU stay. She could last for weeks or months."

Kate dropped her head. Her worst nightmare was coming true. She said, "I can't believe the suffering that she's gone through. She has no prospect of quality life. Only more suffering."

Then Kate looked up and asked, "Have you talked to her son lately?"

"I talked to him yesterday. No changes. I reminded him that I don't believe this is what she wanted. I also talked to him about transferring her to a long-term acute care hospital," said Dr. Dawson.

"Transferring where?" asked Kate with a hint of desperation in her voice.

"It's a private hospital that can provide ventilator support. We can't send a ventilator patient to a nursing home or a skilled nursing facility. Once she's stable, she can't remain here. We need to keep our beds open for acutely ill patients, and she's getting to the point where she doesn't fit that category."

A wave of panic washed over Kate as she realized that Mrs. Pelino might leave Mercy before she died.

While here at Mercy, Kate knew she could help her and ensure her comfort. She wondered what it would be like at the long-term facility and how long Mrs. Pelino might survive in this terrible condition.

Kate felt like time was running out. Mrs. Pelino needed to die according to her wishes, and they were prolonging her dying. Kate thought of the promises she made to Maria Pelino at her bedside. Without a word, Kate turned and left the room.

21

That night Kate met Meg for coffee. There was something different about Kate, but Meg couldn't put her finger on it. Kate almost always seemed relaxed and relieved to sit down with her evening coffee, but on this night, she was distracted. She even fidgeted in her seat and couldn't focus on the conversation, let alone maintain eye contact.

Meg finally asked, "What's up Kate? I've never seen you so jumpy."

Kate was silent for a few seconds and then blurted out, "I'm still really bummed about that stupid mistake I made with that patient."

"The note you forgot to write?"

"Yeah." Kate paused. "She's getting better," she said.

"That's amazing. I thought she didn't have a chance. You doctors are miracle workers," Meg said, hoping to lift Kate's spirits.

Kate shook her head and whispered, "It's no 'miracle.'"

"How can someone like her hold on?"

"The wonders of modern medicine," said Kate, rolling her eyes. "Sometimes we get people well enough to prolong their dying, but not well enough to resume living."

Meg interrupted, "What if you wouldn't have put her on the ventilator?"

Kate dropped her head again. "She would have died peacefully."

Meg sat forward and demanded, "How could someone die peacefully of pneumonia?"

"With Comfort Care, people can die painlessly of pneumonia. Sedatives and narcotics blunt that terrible feeling of breathlessness, and they don't suffer."

"Is that euthanasia?" asked Meg, as her interest grew.

Kate's expression changed. Her anxiety reemerged. She almost looked angry. "No. Euthanasia is illegal here. We don't do that. We can't do that. Doctors don't kill people. We keep people comfortable and let nature take its course. We let people die naturally and relatively pain free with Comfort Care. Everyone has to die sometime, Meg."

Meg didn't understand Kate's angst and asked, "You seem pretty upset by this euthanasia discussion. You didn't think I was accusing you of anything like that, did you?"

Kate took a few deep breaths and settled back in her chair. "I'm just stressed out watching this lady suffer. When I sit at her bedside and try to comfort her, I keep remembering what she told me she wanted. I wish there was more I could do."

"I think you're doing everything you can, Kate. You're helping her," encouraged Meg.

"I wish I could help her have what I know she wants," said Kate.

"To die naturally?"

"Yeah. To die and be at peace."

"Seems as though there's nothing else you can do, but help keep her comfortable," said Meg. "Can you think of anything else?"

Kate shook her head and looked down. "I guess not," she whispered.

22

Kate climbed out of bed the next morning, feeling the sour stomach, itchy eyes, and achy muscles of a sleepless night. She could not shake the self-recrimination and the questions: "Is there anything else I can do? Is there anything else I *should* do?"

The team of residents rounded before meeting up with Dr. Dawson. While in Mrs. Pelino's room, Jack asked, "How's your patient, Dr. DoGood?" with his usual mockery.

"Mrs. Pelino had a temp of 100.8 last night, and I think she might have a urinary tract infection. We need to delay her release," stressed Kate.

"No way, DoGood. She's been on our service long enough, and it's time to go. They can deal with the infection. Start the antibiotics, and we'll send her tomorrow as planned," Jack countered.

Kate knew she couldn't win this battle, so she wrote the orders and tried another approach. Later that day, she appealed to Dr. Dawson, but he agreed with Jack. It was time for Mrs. Pelino to leave Mercy.

That afternoon, Kate checked in on Mrs. Pelino. As usual, the doors were open in most of the ICU rooms. The nurse had drawn the curtain across the door in Mrs. Pelino's room to provide some privacy.

Kate knocked on the door frame, pushed the curtain aside, and sat down at Mrs. Pelino's bedside. She grasped her hand and said, "Hi, Maria."

She opened her eyes and slowly turned toward Kate.

"Are you having any pain?"

She continued to look at Kate with vacant eyes.

Kate looked around the room at the ventilator and all the monitoring equipment, all so carefully designed to keep people alive. Alarms on the ventilator, the EKG, and an oxygen monitor on Mrs. Pelino's finger—all designed to alert the staff of any substantial changes. Once alerted, they could do everything just like Thomas Pelino desired. "'Everything,'" thought Kate. "I wish more people knew the misery of 'everything.'"

Just then, the respiratory therapist darted in to check on Mrs. Pelino's ventilator. He pulled out his stethoscope and listened to her breath sounds. Then he looked up at Kate and said, "She needs to be suctioned."

He turned to the ventilator, pushed a few buttons, then turned back and disconnected Mrs. Pelino from the ventilator. He gently pushed a small tube through the tracheostomy and into the airway to suction the material that Mrs. Pelino was too weak to cough out. Suddenly, the ventilator blared as it sensed the interruption of its circuit. The therapist whirled around, punched in a code, and the alarm died. Then he resumed his work.

After he finished caring for Mrs. Pelino, Kate asked, "Would you mind showing me how that ventilator works? I'm around these things every day, but I don't know much about them."

"Sure, no problem. It's easier than it looks." He quickly provided a crash course in ventilator settings and alarm management.

Kate was on call that night and stopped back to check on Mrs. Pelino. She looked comfortable enough and showed no signs of pain or shortness of breath. Kate noticed that one of the EKG patches was loose and asked the nurse to replace it. She noted where they stored the EKG supplies.

As she walked through the nurse's station, Kate paused to look at the screen that displayed the EKG tracings. An alarm sounded, and the tracing flashed for one of the patients as his heart rate elevated. Kate glanced up to see the nurses comforting the agitated patient. Then she sat down and grabbed the mouse and touched Mrs. Pelino's name, bringing to the display any previous abnormalities. As usual for Mrs. Pelino, a normal rhythm.

Kate's cell phone buzzed—the ER again. She headed out of Mrs. Pelino's room toward the elevator while she answered. She planned to stop back later to check on Mrs. Pelino.

23

ER admissions finally slowed down by 2 a.m., and Kate returned to the ICU. She looked in on Mrs. Pelino, who seemed comfortable. Then she sat at the nurses' station, thumbing through Mrs. Pelino's chart. There was nothing new, but it provided an excuse to sit and observe. The nurses didn't know that Kate had the chart memorized.

Kate watched the nurses as they cared for their patients. The ratio was 2:1, two patients to one nurse. Mrs. Pelino was relatively easy to care for, but that was not so for a few others that night. They already had one code in the ICU, and stress levels among the staff were high.

Nurses and techs were bustling about the room of a man who had just returned from abdominal surgery to deal with a gunshot wound. A drug deal had gone bad, and he took two slugs of lead to the belly. Kate had heard the surgeons discussing the case in the ER.

The guy was lucky. The bullets ripped through his intestines, but missed the major arteries and his spine. If the bullet had hit a major artery, he would have bled to death. If it had hit his spinal cord, he'd be a paraplegic. After surgery, they were having problems keeping his blood pressure up, so he needed close attention.

Kate glanced up as a nurse hustled in and out of Mrs. Pelino's room to suction her airway and provide a dose of sedative before returning to help with the gunshot victim. Kate closed the chart and got up. She took a deep breath and was in Mrs. Pelino's room with a few steps. She drew the curtain across the door and walked to Mrs. Pelino's bedside. The room was dark. The only light came from the monitoring screen above the bed and the street lights four stories down.

Kate sat down and grasped her hand and with the gentle voice of one comforting a friend, Kate asked, "Maria, are you awake?" There was no response, as Kate expected since Mrs. Pelino had just received the sedative. She watched her chest rise and fall with the blowing sound of the ventilator.

Kate sat stroking Maria's hand. She'd never felt so confused. She was bound by law to abide by Thomas Pelino's decisions, but she could not live with the agony of Maria's prolonged dying. She was caught between what she knew was right and what was legally correct.

Kate stared at the EKG monitor tracing across the screen and listened to the whirl of the ventilator. She could hear every sound in the ICU through the thin veil stretched across the doorway. Kate accepted full blame for this mess. A few lines of documentation that day in the clinic would have saved Maria from weeks of suffering and saved enough money to help dozens of people like Toni.

Kate knew she had caused this disaster and was the only one who could fix it.

She rose laboriously, as if lifting Mrs. Pelino on her shoulders, and gazed at Mrs. Pelino's failing form. She swept Maria's hair from her face, leaned forward, and kissed her forehead. Then she whispered in her ear, "I'll give you your wish."

With that, Kate rushed into action. She knew the nurse would be back in about 20 minutes unless she triggered an alarm.

She started with the EKG monitor. Mrs. Pelino's electrode wires converged into a quick-release plug, so Kate grabbed five electrode patches and jerked her scrub top up to affix the patches. She pulled another set of wires with a plug from the drawer and connected the wires to the patches. The wires hung from beneath her green scrub top.

Next she moved to the ventilator. Kate's palms were sweaty and her breathing rapid. The control panel was familiar now thanks to her earlier lesson from the respiratory therapist. She tapped in the code and disabled the alarms.

There was no time to waste. Kate disconnected the ventilator from Mrs. Pelino. Alarms were silenced and Maria's chest was barely moving. Then in a flurry, she disconnected Mrs. Pelino's quick-release plug and connected her own to the EKG monitor. She paused, wondering if the change would trigger an alarm. She heard two tones come from the monitoring station, but that was it. The alarm did not continue.

Now Maria could die in peace. Kate sat down and tried to relax by taking deep slow breaths. She didn't want her own rapid heart rate from the excitement to trigger an alarm. She'd been still for just a few breaths when she glanced up at the monitor. She saw the oxygen levels dropping precipitously, and a short *beep* sounded. Kate gasped.

She'd forgotten the oxygen monitor. She grabbed the plastic clip from Mrs. Pelino's finger, and within seconds, it was on Kate's finger, and only one other *beep* sounded. Kate hoped the nurses were occupied with the other patients and would not investigate.

She heard footsteps. They sounded like boulders rolling down the corridor as someone passed the room.

Kate took deep slow breaths and closed her eyes, making every effort to relax. She watched her heart rate climb to 125 and knew the alarm would sound at 130. She battled her own nervous system and won as her heart rate receded to less than 120.

Kate held Maria's hand and monitored her pulse with the gentle touch of an index finger over the artery in Maria's wrist. Maria's chest barely moved and stopped completely within two minutes of being off the ventilator.

Her heart continued to pump, but she was not able to provide adequate oxygen to her heart, brain, and other tissues. Her pulse was barely palpable at two minutes. By four minutes, it was gone. Kate placed her stethoscope in her ears and listened for heart sounds for the next two minutes—there were none. Kate knew that Mrs. Pelino was now clinically dead but also knew that patients with no respirations and an absent pulse could still be revived, so she waited and sweated. Kate took more deep breaths and closed her eyes as she saw her heart rate inching above 120 again. "Just relax," she thought, "This is almost over."

When Kate removed the stethoscope, she heard two people talking. Her senses were so activated that she could hear every syllable, as if they were right beside her. She hoped they were too busy to check on Mrs. Pelino. Kate's heart rate was over 120 again. She covered her ears and closed her eyes and forced her heart rate to 110.

Mrs. Pelino was limp and pale after being pulseless for 10 minutes. Her hand was cool. Her lips and fingers were a bluish gray like a drab winter sky. But she was finally at peace. Kate forced herself to wait longer; there must not be any chance for a successful Code. Just the thought of resuscitating Mrs. Pelino caused a wave of nausea to flush through Kate, especially knowing what was coming.

Kate glanced at her watch and the EKG monitor. Her pulse was down to 113. She took more deep, slow breaths and closed her eyes. The vivid memory of her first meeting with Maria gave her courage to carry on. Kate knew this is what Maria wanted. She looked at the thin curtain, hoping that no one would enter. Someone dropped a chart on the floor, and it sounded like a thunderbolt. Kate winced as her pulse quickened again. She fought the adrenaline surge that might trigger an alarm. Finally 20 minutes had passed. The nurse would return soon. Mrs. Pelino was gone. She was at peace. She had died naturally. She would feel no pain. It was time for the next move.

Kate placed Mrs. Pelino back on the ventilator and reactivated the alarms. She made sure all the settings were correct. The ventilator was working, and Mrs. Pelino's chest was moving, but she was gone. The next step had to occur quickly because the alarms would trigger immediately.

In a flash, Kate reattached Mrs. Pelino to the EKG monitor and placed the oxygen monitor back on her finger. She looked at the EKG monitor—flat line. Now the acting would have to begin. "It was all for Maria's good," she kept reminding herself. "Mrs. Pelino is gone. This won't hurt her now."

In a flurry, Kate removed the patches and EKG electrodes from her own chest and tossed them in the trash can, covering them with some paper. Then she rushed out of the room. The EKG alarm was blaring. Kate ran toward the nurses' station and shouted, "Call a Code for Mrs. Pelino in Room 5011." *Ping, ping, ping: Code Blue Room 5011.*

Kate returned and started chest compressions with one of the nurses. She tried to be gentle but still felt Mrs. Pelino's ribs snap under her weight. The rest of the Code team streamed in, and they went through the usual rounds of medications with no results. They followed the protocol precisely and stopped the Code when she failed to respond. Kate pronounced Mrs. Pelino dead. She wrote a brief note that summarized the Code and documented Mrs. Pelino's death at 2:38 a.m.

Maria could finally have the peace she wanted. Kate didn't look forward to calling Thomas Pelino.

As Kate left the ICU, the nurses continued their meticulous documentation. Mrs. Pelino's nurse grabbed several paper strips that the EKG and oxygen monitor had spit out that night and taped them into the chart. By sunrise, the chart was on a shelf in the medical records department.

24

The phone rang, and Kate hoped Thomas Pelino wouldn't answer. When he finally did, he sounded drowsy. It was almost 3 a.m. Kate started, "Mr. Pelino, this is Dr. Simon from Mercy Hospital."

"Yes, what's wrong?" he asked flatly.

"I'm sorry to tell you that your mother's heart stopped, and she died this morning."

"Oh, no," he gasped. "What happened?"

Lies didn't come easily to Kate, but she would have to learn quickly to get through this ordeal. "We're not sure what happened. It looks like her heart suddenly stopped, and we could not resuscitate her."

"Did you do everything you could to save her?"

"We did everything, Mr. Pelino," Kate said. Her heart was pounding, and she felt like running as far from Mercy as she could get. She continued, "Would you like to come in and see her before we move her?"

"Of course. Don't move her. I'll be right in," he snapped.

"I'm sorry, sir. We won't move her." Then Kate asked, "Do you have other questions?"

"Not now." He paused for a few seconds and with the tone of a man pronouncing a curse said, "I guess you and Dr. Dawson got your wish."

Kate stood transfixed because he was right. She recovered and said, "I'm sorry for your loss. If you have other questions, we'll—"

"I'll bet you're sorry," Mr. Pelino fired back and hung up.

Kate sat silently for several minutes by the phone, wondering how this man, who abandoned his mom for 10 years, could do so much damage to his mother in such a short period of time. She shook it off and turned to the next task—a call to Dr. Dawson.

The call was brief and to the point. Dr. Dawson expected Mrs. Pelino to die sooner or later, so it was no surprise. Kate told Dr. Dawson that Mrs. Pelino had gone asystolic and they were unable to resuscitate her. She also filled him in on the conversation with Mr. Pelino. Dr. Dawson said, "I'm glad she's at peace. I'll see you in a few hours," and hung up. Kate was glad to have that behind her.

At around 5 a.m., the ICU called. "Mr. Pelino is here to see you." Kate fought back cresting waves of nausea as she walked down the hall. She entered Mrs. Pelino's room, and he was at the bedside. His eyes were moist, but anger, not sorrow, flooded his face. "How could you let this happen to my mother?" he shouted.

"Mr. Pelino, your mother's heart stopped. We were unable to resuscitate her. We did everything we could." Kate continued, "Do you have any questions?"

"I don't have any questions. I just want to get my mother out of here."

"The chaplain is here, and she can help you with all the arrangements," said Kate, as she turned to the young woman outside the door. "I'll leave you with her, and if you have other questions, the nurses can call me."

Mr. Pelino never looked at Kate again and stood silently beside the bed as she walked out of the room. The bright red glow of the rising September sun struck Kate through the window.

25

Kate hurried to the call room, took a quick shower, and put on a fresh set of scrubs. She found that by getting a shower she could fool her body and mind into thinking she had gotten some sleep. She was exhausted, yet relieved, knowing that Mrs. Pelino was at peace. She had helped her end her life in comfort and with dignity. No more needless suffering. No more needless expenditures. What a relief. But Kate was feeling troubled by the prospect of living with this secret.

She looked in on her patients and went to meet up with the team in the ICU. Jack greeted her. "Good morning, Dr. DoGood. I see your patient died last night."

Kate tried to remain expressionless and said, "She went asystolic. We couldn't get her back."

"You must be pretty happy."

"Not happy, but I'm glad she's not suffering." Kate kept looking at a chart, avoiding eye contact. She wondered if Jack suspected anything.

Dr. Dawson joined them, and Kate was relieved that nothing else was mentioned about Mrs. Pelino's case. She was surprised that Jack let the issue rest.

As they were ending their morning rounds, Dr. Dawson pulled Kate aside and said, "I know this has been really tough on you. You did your best, and I don't want to see that one documentation mistake ruin your life. You need to be easier on yourself. We all make mistakes, Kate."

Kate stood in silence.

"You've experienced a terrible, prolonged death. I'd like you to get another perspective, if you're interested."

Kate looked up. "What did you have in mind?"

"You met Brian Richardson, a hospice nurse, a few weeks ago. I saw him this morning, and he agreed to let you tag along with him. Would you like to do that?"

Kate showed no emotion. Then she said, "That sounds good. When can I go?"

"Will tomorrow afternoon work?"

"That's fine, Dr. Dawson."

"I'll have Brian meet you in the hospital lobby about noon. I need to get to the office now," he said as he hurried away, leaving Kate standing in the corridor.

26

Around noon the next day, Kate finished her work and rushed to the elevator. She had met Brian Richardson, the hospice nurse, one time. She wondered what made someone want to deal with dying patients every day. She looked forward to getting out of the hospital and as far from Jack as possible. She knew it was probably paranoia but couldn't shake the sense that Jack suspected her in Maria's death.

Brian met her with a big smile as she stepped off the elevator into the lobby. His full head of gray hair reminded Kate of her grandfather. Brian thrust his hand forward and said, "Good to see you again, Dr. Simon."

"Good to see you, Brian. Please call me Kate."

"Okay, Kate. Let's get rolling. We need to get to Maple Manor to evaluate a nursing home patient by 12:30. He has severe dementia, and his family is considering hospice care."

Brian motioned toward the front door and led the way to his car. As he opened the door, he said, "Sorry for all the mess. This is my office and supply center." The back seat was piled high with papers and medical supplies. Packages of bandages and syringes cascaded down the mountain of boxes.

Kate rolled her eyes. "No problem, Brian. You should see my car." They both laughed.

As they pulled away from Mercy, Brian asked, "What do you know about hospice, Kate?"

"I know hospice provides care for patients in their last days of life, emphasizing Comfort Care, but that's about it."

"Our main mission is outside the hospital. Not that hospitals are bad, of course," he said with a playful grin. "But when people get to the point where their disease is no longer responsive to life-prolonging therapy, then it's time to change the goals. That's why, in most cases, hospitalization is not part of hospice care."

Brian continued, "The goal of hospice is to improve the quality of a patient's last days by offering comfort and dignity. In most cases, that's best done in their home or a nursing home."

"We offer comfort and dignity in the hospital," retorted Kate, a bit defensively.

"Of course you do, Kate. I'm not saying hospital care is bad, but I think you'll see a difference. Then you'll know why people want to stay out of the hospital and die in peace with their family at their own bedside."

"I understand. Tell me how hospice started."

"Well, it was Dr. Cicely Saunders who got it going. She opened a place called St. Christopher's in England in 1967. They had just 40 beds, but it was a peaceful place for people to go when they were dying. They gave people a chance to care for their loved ones as they died."

"What's the main advantage of hospice?"

"We have a team of professionals who care for the patient and the family. Hospice care of the family continues after the patient's death to help them grieve well."

"Tell me more about pain control."

"Hospice physicians pioneered the use of pain management to actually relieve pain. Physicians tend to be reluctant to prescribe higher doses of narcotic analgesics that terminal patients often need to manage pain. Most cancer patients died with excruciating pain before the hospice movement."

"Do patients get pain relief today?"

"I think most hospice patients do, but I've met many patients outside hospice care who were undermedicated and experienced agonizing pain until we got involved."

"Why's that happen?"

"Some physicians are not experienced with pain control in terminal illness, and they fear overdosing patients. But realize, there are many non-hospice physicians who understand pain control and do an excellent job."

"Is hospice only for cancer patients?"

Brian shook his head as he sped down the exit ramp. "We care for anyone who has a terminal illness and has decided they don't want to pursue life-prolonging treatments. Patients with all kinds of diseases, including those with heart and lung disease, are well served by hospice. Many of our patients have Alzheimer's disease or other causes of severe dementia."

"I didn't know that."

"It's a common misunderstanding, Kate. I wish more doctors and patients realized what we offer. They'd find that we could help them enjoy their last days with their family and die with peace and dignity in their home in most cases." He continued, "Patients who live in nursing homes can benefit from hospice, too. In fact, that's where we'll begin today."

Both fell silent. Kate couldn't get Maria and Mrs. Frank out of her mind. She cringed while remembering the sensations of shattering ribs. She had to remind herself again that she did everything she could to help Maria die with peace and dignity.

When they arrived at the nursing home, Brian said, "We received a referral for a patient with severe dementia whose family wants to consider hospice."

As they walked into the lobby, the receptionist said, "Hi Brian. Who are you here to see today?"

"Hello, Helen. It's nice to see you. We're here to see Kevin Foster on the Alzheimer's Unit."

"Okay, Brian. You can go ahead, but be careful. One of the patients has been trying to escape all morning. I'll wait until you get close to the door to unlock it."

Brian led the way to a large wooden door with a small plate-glass window in the middle. He peered through the window and nodded toward Helen. She buzzed the door, and Brian pushed through.

Brian turned to Kate and said, "Looks like the coast is clear. No escape attempts."

Kate looked confused. "Escape attempts?"

"Patients on this unit have severe dementia. They have no short-term memory, and many can't recall distant memories either. Some are still physically fit, and sometimes they try to get out. That's why it's locked."

When they turned the corner of the tiled hallway, there were two patients sitting in rolling recliners. Both had pillows under their right shoulder, propping them on one side. Neither noticed Brian and Kate as they strolled past, but Kate stopped and knelt on one knee beside the frail woman's chair and looked straight into her eyes. Kate glanced at her ID bracelet and then said, "Hello, Mrs. Woods."

A hint of a smile grew ever so slowly on the woman's wrinkled face. Her eyes were sunken, and her skin clung to her facial bones. Kate remembered the skull she studied in med school as she inspected the woman's features.

"How are you today, Mrs. Woods?"

The smile persisted, but an answer did not come. Kate waited patiently for several seconds, then squeezed her hand and stood up. "Goodbye, Mrs. Woods."

Kate's eyes met Brian's and she said, "Getting old is tough."

"Sure is." Brian pointed to the next door. "Here's Mr. Foster's room."

Brian knocked on the open door. "Brian Richardson from hospice here."

A man's voice answered, "Come in."

A woman and man, both of retirement age, sat in two over-stuffed chairs beside the window. The colors were warm, and the sun shone through the large window. A Monet print hung alongside the bed, and oak furniture appointed the room. About a dozen family pictures stood on the bookshelf, and three more sat on the bedside table. One showed a large family with two older, fit-appearing folks sitting in the middle. Mr. Foster was curled up in the bed on his right side, facing toward the room. The covers were pulled up to his chin so that only his head was visible. Like the woman in the hall, his face was thin. He moved only slightly as they entered the room.

Both people rose to greet Brian and Kate.

The gentleman stuck out his hand and said, "I'm Bill Foster, his son, and this is my sister, Mae Glen."

"Nice to meet you. I'm Brian Richardson and this is Dr. Kate Simon. She's working with me today and is a physician-in-training at Mercy. How's your father doing?"

"He seems fine, except he's been sleepier recently."

Brian said, "I'd like to start by examining him, and then we can discuss hospice."

Brian pulled a chair alongside the bed and leaned toward Mr. Foster's face. He said, "Mr. Foster can you hear me?"

He opened his eyes and whispered, "Yes."

"Can you tell me your name?"

"Kevin Foster."

"Do you know where you are?"

"I'm at the store."

"Do you know the date or the year?"

He hesitated and his eyes darted, then he said, "I'm not sure, but I think it's 1978."

"Who are these two people?"

He was brightening up as he answered the questions. He lifted his head to look across the room. "I need my glasses to see them."

Brian laughed and said, "I'm sorry, Mr. Foster." He grabbed the glasses from the table and placed them on Mr. Foster's nose.

He looked intently at his two children and said, "They look familiar, but I don't know them. I'm glad they're visiting me." He smiled.

Kate glanced at Mrs. Glen and saw a tear well in her eye. She pulled a tissue from her purse and dabbed her eye.

Brian turned toward the two and asked, "How long's it been since he's known you?"

"About a year and a half," answered Mr. Foster. "He's been a wonderful father, and it's so difficult watching him waste away like this."

"Has he had other medical problems recently?"

"He's had pneumonia three times in the last six months and a urinary tract infection just last month."

"Was he hospitalized for those conditions?"

"Yes."

"So he's been to the hospital four times in the last six months, right?"

"That's right," said Mr. Foster. "Every hospital visit is hard on him. He's accustomed to life here, and he gets disoriented in the hospital. He needs restraints to keep him in bed and sometimes he needs sedatives." He looked at his sister and back to Brian and said, "We think we're not doing the best thing for Dad by sending him back and forth to treat these conditions. We need help."

Brian kept eye contact and nodded. "We can help you. The philosophy behind hospice is to provide Comfort Care and allow people to die without pain and with dignity. We have a team of professionals that can work with you and the nursing home staff to care for your dad."

"That's what we're looking for. Dad would not want to live this way. He was always active and full of life. We hate to see him suffer."

"Our goal is comfort, and we could do that here or in a home. If you agree to the hospice approach, we would not hospitalize your dad unless we could not keep him comfortable. We would not treat any conditions to prolong his life."

"What would happen if he develops pneumonia or a urinary tract infection?" asked Mrs. Glen.

"We would not hospitalize him, and we would only prescribe antibiotics if he needed them to enhance his comfort."

"We've been talking about this, and we definitely want to take the hospice approach for the rest of Dad's life," said Mr. Foster. His sister nodded in agreement.

"We'll need you to sign a few papers and also talk to your dad's doctor to get an order for Do Not Resuscitate and Do Not Hospitalize."

Mr. Foster moved forward on his chair and asked, "Could we have decided to not hospitalize Dad earlier, or did we need hospice for that?"

"Any patient or their designated decision maker can refuse life-prolonging care. You could have made that decision at any time."

Mr. Foster wrung his hands. He looked at his sister and asked her, "Did you know that, Mae?"

"I remember some mention of that when Dad was admitted here about five years ago, but frankly I forgot."

Mr. Foster shook his head.

Brian asked, "Has the issue come up since then?"

"No, sir," said Mr. Foster. His jaw tightened as he stared at his father. He looked at his sister and said, "Mae, we should have done this a year ago. This last year has been so hard on Dad, and his quality of life has been awful."

"You're right, but we were trying to do the best thing. We've never been through this before," she said.

Brian interrupted, "Now we know what you want, and we'll take care of him. We'll help keep him comfortable."

Mr. Foster took a deep breath and said, "Thanks, Brian. That will be a great relief to Dad."

Brian finished the paperwork and bid farewell. He phoned the physician to change the Code status and establish the Do Not Hospitalize status before they left. Then they walked to the car and headed toward their next stop.

Brian was silent as they traveled. His eyes were fixed straight ahead, and his face was tense.

After a few minutes, Kate couldn't stand the silence. "What's bothering you, Brian?"

He cleared his throat, took a deep breath, and said, "I can't get used to seeing people like Mr. Foster suffer through their last months of life. Look how he and his family have agonized through this last year." He stopped and glanced at Kate.

She nodded. "Is the problem limited to this part of the country?"

Brian shook his head and with more than a hint of sarcasm he said, "I wish it was. There was a study published in 2007 that looked at how we deal with patients who have severe dementia. Patients like

Mr. Foster. You would expect that most patients like Mr. Foster, who are severely demented, would not be treated aggressively and would have Do Not Hospitalize orders, right?"

"Of course! It's clearly not in their best interest to go to a hospital unless they couldn't provide adequate Comfort Care."

"That's right. Here's what the nationwide study found. Only seven percent of patients with severe dementia in nursing homes have a Do Not Hospitalize order." Brian paused to let the fact settle in. He continued, "That means 93 percent of patients with severe dementia, who are nursing home residents, are transported to hospitals when they become ill. We prolong dying in these patients. They suffer needlessly, and I can't imagine the financial burden. It's a tragic waste. Almost all of them would be better served with Comfort Care, either at home or in a nursing home."

"Do you think all severely demented patients should automatically be DNR and Do Not Hospitalize?"

"Absolutely not! We don't want to take decision making out of people's hands. I wish more people would get the education they need to make good end-of-life decisions. Just like Mr. Foster's children. Clearly, no one educated them or gave them the DNR/Do Not Hospitalize option in recent months."

"What can I do?"

"When patients come into the hospital, you can be sure they and their families know their options. If they change their status to DNR, communicate that to the nursing home. If they want to change to Do Not Hospitalize, too, then they need to take that up with the nursing home staff."

"I'll try."

Brian glanced toward Kate, a bit bewildered. "What makes you so interested?"

"I've had a few cases already where patients really suffered at the end of life, and I want to do whatever I can to prevent that agony for others."

Kate fell silent. She thought about Maria and wondered if anyone suspected her in the death. She didn't want to provide clues to anyone, including Brian.

Brian interrupted the silence. "I've met a lot of young doctors, and frankly there aren't many that care about what happens as death approaches. What makes you care about these people?"

Kate pondered the question. "It's probably the way I was raised."

"Would you mind telling me about that?"

"Not at all. When I was eight, we moved to Cambodia. Dad was a physician and Mom was a nurse. We grew up among people with unbelievable needs, and they were so thankful for the simple things we could give.

"Mom and Dad always put my sister and me to work in the clinic, and we loved it. That's where I fell in love with medicine and learned about caring for people."

"Is your sister a doctor, too?"

"No. She hates blood. And other body fluids." They both laughed.

"My sister was always more interested in administration and organization. She has her MBA and works in banking now. When I finish my residency, we plan to move back to Cambodia. It's really our home. I'll work in the clinic, and my sister wants to help build the micro-lending network."

"Wow. You two are unusual. Your parents must be proud."

Kate fell silent for several seconds. Then she said, "They would be."

Brian glanced her way. "Are they gone?"

"They died about three years ago in a plane crash. Every week they traveled to a remote village for a clinic, and they got into bad weather." Kate looked down at the floor.

"I'm so sorry, Kate."

"It's been really hard for my sister and me, but she moved here too, and we help each other. I've been missing my parents a lot lately."

Kate wondered if she'd be in this mess if she had Mom and Dad to talk to.

Brian said, "I'm sure your parents would be proud of you."

The statement rattled Kate. She considered whether they'd be proud of what she'd done, but she couldn't discuss that with Brian.

With a forced sense of poise she said, "They'd be proud of me. You could never find two people more committed to caring for needy people. So I guess that's where some, if not all, of my sense of caring comes from."

The memories flooded in, washing a wave of relief over Kate. A smile broke across her face. "Some days hundreds of people would line up outside our clinic. We all worked hard. Dad and Mom also trained Cambodian doctors and nurses. You can't imagine the impact they had."

They both sat silently, and then Kate said, "I've always wanted to be like them. Thanks for asking me about my family. It's painful, but I enjoy the memories."

"Thanks for your openness. You've had quite a rich life."

Brian pointed ahead and said, "Our next stop is just around the corner."

27

They had just entered a neighborhood of well-kept, 1930s-era homes, equipped with large front porches. Mature trees lined the streets. Flowers bloomed and lawns were green. They pulled along the curb in front of a two-story white house with red shutters. Roses bloomed along the front porch where two women sat.

"This is Mr. Steve Mallory's home. He has end-stage lung disease. That's his daughter and sister on the porch," he said, nodding their way.

When they hopped out of the car, the two women jumped up. The younger one shouted, "Hi, Brian." Brian waved, and the two scurried down the steps to meet their visitors.

"This is Dr. Kate Simon. She's training to be a family physician at Mercy and is interested in hospice care."

"So nice to meet you. I'm Connie, Steve's daughter."

"And I'm his sister, Krystal. Come on in."

Brian held the door as the three women entered. They made their way into a dining room dominated by a large oak table covered with pieces of a jigsaw puzzle. Mr. Mallory tilted his head up and looked over his glasses as they entered the room. He smiled when he saw Brian pop around the corner.

He was seated and leaning over the table with his elbows resting on the table. With each breath, his neck muscles contracted as he labored to draw enough air to sustain his life. A plastic tube carried oxygen from a tank in the corner to two prongs that rested in his nostrils. Kate noticed calluses on his elbows from the years spent bracing himself with his arms to get air.

"It's good to see you out of bed," said Brian, as if he were greeting his best friend.

Mr. Mallory took a few deep breaths and said, "Took a lot..." he took a few more breaths and continued, "...of effort to get here." He stopped and gasped for air.

Brian gripped his shoulder. "You don't need to say anything, Steve. I'll ask some questions, and you just shake your head.

"Are you making any progress on this puzzle?"

Steve smiled and nodded, pointing to the border he'd assembled.

"Nice work." Brian pointed toward Kate. "This is Dr. Simon. She's along for the afternoon, so she can learn about hospice."

He nodded toward Kate and smiled as he drew another breath.

Brian pulled out his stethoscope and listened over Steve's back. Then he handed it to Kate and pointed to Steve. After she was done, Brian asked, "What did you hear?"

"Hardly any breath sounds. No wheezing or rhonchi."

Brian nodded. "That's right. His lung tissue is mostly gone. He has severe emphysema."

Mr. Mallory took a few big gasps and whispered, "Too many cigarettes."

Brian asked, "Have you been sleeping okay?"

He shook his head, no.

"Coughing?"

He nodded, yes.

"Remember the cough medicine I left? Don't forget to take it." Brian turned toward the women and said, "Make sure he gets the cough syrup at bedtime. He can have another dose during the night if the cough wakes him up.

"Are you feeling any pain or anxiety?" asked Brian.

Steve shook his head and said, "Medicine's…working." He needed one breath for each word, but he managed a smile.

His daughter chimed in. "The change you suggested in the pain medicine has really helped with his back pain and the feeling of suffocation. His breathing is labored, but he's not uncomfortable."

They heard the back door open, and within moments, a portly black lab bounded into the room and Mrs. Fran Mallory followed. The dog greeted the new guests, and then went to Steve's side where he sat and laid his head on Steve's thigh. Steve stroked him and whispered, "Hi, Duke." Duke's tail continued to swing as he eyed the guests, but he remained by his master.

"Hello, Fran. Steve's updating us right now. He told us that he's been coughing, but the pain and anxiety are better. Any other problems?" asked Brian.

"I'm worried about his appetite. He's skin and bones and getting skinnier by the day," said Fran with a look of deep concern.

Brian moved toward her side of the table and pulled out a chair for her. They both sat down, and Brian looked straight into her eyes. "In the end stages of this disease, people usually lose their appetite."

"I remember you said that before, but I hate to see him wasting away."

"I understand. Our goal is to keep him comfortable, and if forcing food and liquids causes discomfort, then we don't want to push it." Brian turned toward Steve and asked, "Are you hungry or thirsty?"

Steve shook his head, no.

Fran looked down at the table. The room grew silent except for Steve's respirations. Then she looked up at Brian with misty eyes and said, "I don't think he can live long without eating."

Brian took her hand and looked back and forth at the two of them. "I know this is really difficult, but you and your family are doing what Steve wants. Never forget that. He decided that he did not want any care that would prolong his dying. He wants only Comfort Care, and we are all committed to respecting his wishes."

Fran nodded in agreement, as a tear rolled down her cheek.

Brian squeezed her hand and she looked up. When their eyes met, he said, "You, your family, and friends are doing an awesome job." He turned to Steve. "You're facing your future with courage, Steve."

She wrapped her arm around Steve and pulled him close. He smiled between labored breaths.

Brian asked, "Is there anything else I can do to help?"

Fran said, "Could you send the chaplain by again? She comforted us and read the Bible to us. She prayed with us, and I sensed a weight lifted from Steve after she was here yesterday."

"I'll call her when we leave." Brian looked into the backyard and said, "It's beautiful today. How would you like to sit in the sun?"

Steve's smile was bigger than ever as he nodded.

His daughter pushed the wheelchair alongside his chair, and Brian helped Fran scoot him over. His daughter carried the oxygen tank while Brian pushed him through the back door, down the ramp, and onto the deck. The sky was clear blue, and the sun burned brilliantly. Steve's chin lifted and his respirations seemed to ease a little, as the sun struck his face. Brian locked the wheels and stood back.

Kate watched as the dog plodded down the ramp and curled up at Steve's feet. Then his family drew around him. A breeze stirred the trees, and a robin settled by the flower bed. Kate imagined Steve tending the garden and realized the joy he must have, here in his own backyard, looking at the garden he created.

She'd forgotten that Brian was beside her, but now she watched him from the corner of her eye and saw a satisfied smile spread across his face. She hoped that she would be able to have the same satisfaction of caring for people that she saw in him.

"Anything else we can do today?" asked Brian.

Fran shook her head. "No. You'll never know how much we appreciate you and the rest of the hospice team." The others, including Steve, nodded in agreement.

"We're glad to help." Brian bid farewell and strolled up the ramp and back through the house. He stopped in the dining room and stared out the window at Steve, his family, and his dog, all basking in the sun.

His jaw tightened ever so slightly as he pointed toward the deck and said, "You'll never see that in the hospital, Kate." He took a deep breath and sighed while heading toward the front door and down the steps toward the car. He seemed lost in his thoughts.

As they pulled away, Brian called the chaplain for the Mallory family, and then he asked Kate, "What did you think of your first hospice home visit?"

Kate sat silently for several seconds. "Peaceful...yeah, peaceful. Even though he was gasping for air, he had peace. Being in his home, being cared for by his family made all the difference in the world. Having Duke at his side seemed to make his dying more tolerable, too."

"Was it different than watching someone die in the hospital?"

Kate swallowed hard. She saw Brian glance her way. She knew Brian didn't know Maria, but still his question rattled her. She fought to keep composed.

"Yeah. His experience of dying is much different than what I've seen so far." Kate grew silent as she thought of the stark contrast between the experiences of Maria and Steve. She thought of Mrs. Frank, too.

The silence unnerved Kate. Finally she asked, "Why don't more people choose hospice?"

"I don't think they know it's an option. Most people think it's just for cancer patients. Besides, physicians are trained to save lives, and I don't think our education system does a very good job helping doctors know when to advise end-of-life care. If doctors don't suggest hospice, then it usually doesn't get done. In some cases, patients or families request hospice, but that's an exception."

Kate nodded and sat quietly.

Brian brightened and said, "I'm glad to see that cynicism and a cold heart aren't your problems." He glanced at Kate and she smiled but said nothing. Brian continued, "It's easy to grow cold as a medical professional."

She shook her head and said, "I hope that never happens to me."

Neither spoke for the next few minutes. She knew Brian would understand her decision to help Maria and wanted to tell him the whole story, but knew she must not.

They pulled up to the hospital, and Kate hopped out. "Thanks, Brian. I learned a lot today, and it was good to get out of the hospital, too." They shook hands and said goodbye.

Kate hurried into the hospital and headed straight to the eighth floor to check on a few patients. When she got off the elevator, Dr. Dawson and Jack were talking in the hallway.

She avoided eye contact, hoping to steer clear of Jack.

Dr. Dawson saw Kate and called, "Kate, seeing you reminded me of something important."

Kate turned back and approached the two physicians.

Dr. Dawson said, "I received a letter from the Quality Review Committee about Mrs. Pelino's unexpected death."

Kate gulped but kept cool. She took a deep, slow breath.

He turned toward Jack. "I'd like you to review the chart, Jack, and see if there was anything we might have missed. Look it over carefully and report back to us next week."

Jack said, "No problem, Dr. Dawson. I'll have it done by Monday."

Kate fidgeted but refused to look at Jack. She thought he was staring at her.

Kate took a deep breath. "Is there anything I need to do, Dr. Dawson?"

"No, Kate. You can just relax. You did enough for Mrs. Pelino, already. Jack can take care of the chart review."

Kate's mouth was dry and her hands were wet. "Thanks, Dr. Dawson. I'll be interested to see what Jack finds."

Dr. Dawson hurried off. Kate turned and walked away from Jack. As she was walking away, Jack said, "You can bet I'll do a careful review, Simon."

28

As soon as Kate was out of Jack's view, she called the medical records department and requested Maria Pelino's chart. It would be available in an hour, so she went to dinner but wasn't hungry. Her head spun as she thought about what a thorough chart review might reveal. Would there be an EKG tracing she hadn't seen? Would someone notice the changes in heart rate while Kate wore the electrodes?

When Kate went to the medical records department, the clerk presented her with a four-inch-thick mass of paper that contained the facts of Mrs. Pelino's hospital course. Kate's palms were wet, and her heart was racing, as she sat down to examine the chart. She knew practically every page, but she wondered what might have appeared at the end. She had forgotten about those records until Dr. Dawson mentioned the chart review.

Kate went straight to the last day. She found her progress note that described the Code and declaration of death. Then she reviewed the Code records that nursing kept. There were no problems so far.

Next she turned to the monitor tracings the nurses had taped into the chart. She shuffled through reams of tracings to get to the end. When she opened to the last page of tracings, her mouth went dry and her pulse raced. The differences between Mrs. Pelino's EKG pattern and Kate's couldn't be more obvious. No one could miss it. She closed the chart and looked over her shoulder.

Kate stood up with the chart and made her way to one of the cubicles in the corner. She covered the chart with a few others that had been left out and walked across the hall to the ER. Kate figured the ER to be the most chaotic place and therefore the best place to get what she needed without arousing suspicion. She managed to give two nurses a carefree greeting as her eyes darted about looking for a tape dispenser. She found one and stuffed it into the pocket of her lab coat.

As she headed for the door, she heard Jack's voice, "Hey Simon, I need some help with a central line in here. I wondered where you were."

Kate's blood ran cold. She stopped and slowly turned around. "I'll be right back. I'm not feeling well, and I need to go to the bathroom."

"You looked fine a few minutes ago."

"This hit me suddenly. I'm sorry, but I need to go." Kate turned and sped out the door.

She knew Jack was busy, so she went straight to the chart. She sat in a secluded cubicle well out of the clerk's sight. There were five strips that she would have to carefully remove, and then she'd reposition the others. First she removed the three EKG tracings: one recording the change in EKG when she placed the leads on herself, another while she wore the leads, and finally a tracing that caught the change back to Mrs. Pelino.

There were also two oxygen monitor tracings that she had to remove. One showed the abrupt drop in oxygen level and then a rapid reversal when Kate placed the monitor on herself. The next one showed excellent oxygen levels right up to the point of cardiac arrest and then a precipitous drop. That correlated with Kate placing the clip back on Mrs. Pelino's finger at the end. Jack or any other savvy physician would be suspicious if he saw these tracings.

Within a few minutes, Kate removed the key tracings and repositioned the others up to fill the spaces. She taped them in place and gave the chart a final inspection. Then she returned it to the clerk and ran to the ER. Her heart was pounding.

She walked to the room where she had left Jack. He was gowned and gloved. He looked up and said, "You're too late, Simon. We needed to get this line in, so I did it myself. There's another patient we need to see in 56. Go get started." Jack went back to work on the patient, and Kate breathed a sigh of relief.

29

Kate was agitated when she left the hospital that evening. On the way home, she called Meg to arrange a run. They met at their usual spot in the park and took off after some quick stretches.

"You seem depressed since that whole thing came down with that patient, Kate."

"It's depressing. I made some bad decisions that are hard to live with." For a moment, Kate nearly blurted out everything that happened with Maria Pelino but caught herself. She wanted Meg to know everything but could not bear to drag her into the mess.

"You've had some tough things happen, Kate. You lost that young woman to poverty and now this recent disaster with the guilty son. I'd be depressed, too."

"I wish I could talk to Mom and Dad." Tears began rolling down Kate's face. She ran faster and Meg kept up.

She continued, "I feel like I wouldn't be in this predicament if they were here."

"What do you mean?"

Kate realized that she'd said more than she intended. "I mean, I wouldn't be so depressed if they were here to talk to."

"It's so different without them," said Meg.

"I've been thinking a lot about Mom lately and our time in Cambodia. Do you remember when we were hiding that young woman in the clinic? She was fleeing from the brothel owner."

"Only vaguely," said Meg. Kate was running faster, and Meg said, "Hey, slow down. I can't keep up."

Kate was skimming along with ease as she told the story, remembering it like it happened yesterday. She recalled being in the back room of the clinic when a young man confronted her mother. He demanded to know the whereabouts of a woman that had run away from the brothel his father operated. He said he knew she was hiding in the clinic and she was worth a lot of money since she was young and beautiful.

Kate's spirits lifted as the memories flowed forth. She remembered their mom telling him that no one has the right to own another person. Then she could hear his growling voice in reply and his threat to return with a knife if their mom refused to cooperate. Kate recounted the quaking in their mom's voice, as she demanded he leave. Kate remembered the fear, and yet, their mom did not give in.

Kate smiled. "When he finally left, I ran into the room and threw my arms around Mom. Ever since that day, I've tried to be that kind of person."

"What do you mean, Kate?"

"I want to be the kind of person who stands up for what they believe in and looks out for others. Especially for people who need help like that woman did."

"There aren't many people like her," said Meg.

"I want to be that way."

"You are, Kate. You need to give yourself a break."

"I'm not very good at that. The perils of being a perfectionist, I guess." They both laughed and their spirits lifted.

They ran in silence for a mile or so, and then Kate said, "I got to see patients with a hospice nurse today, and it was pretty cool."

Kate explained hospice and the visits she'd made with Brian.

Meg asked, "What did you like about hospice?"

"It may sound weird, but it was refreshing to see people face the end of life with courage and realism, rather than pretending that life will go on forever."

They wound down their run as the sun was setting. Kate fought back the urge to spill the truth about Maria. She'd never kept a secret from Meg.

30

Later that week, Kate met up with Dr. Joshua Slone. As one of Dr. Dawson's partners, he was supervising the Internal Medicine team that day. Dr. Slone trained at Mercy and had been on staff for two years. His boyish face raised frequent questions about his credentials, but his confidence and relaxed demeanor put patients at ease.

As Kate approached, he said, "Hello, Kate. Let's get started. Jack will be along later."

Kate followed Dr. Slone to Room 4023. He knocked on the door and said, "Mr. Lutz, Dr. Slone here. Okay to come in?"

"No problem. Come on in," said Mr. Homer Lutz with a chuckle. He had ruddy cheeks and a whopping nose. His broad shoulders and bulky forearms betrayed many years of hard work on the farm, but these days his sons did most of the work. At age 78, he was finally slowing down. His wife, Elaine, sat at the bedside.

After introducing himself, Dr. Slone reviewed Mr. Lutz's history and found that he injured his leg while splitting wood. A sizable shard smashed into his leg, and he developed an infection. He came to the hospital with a swollen red leg, fever, and severe pain.

Dr. Slone examined him carefully, giving special attention to the swelling and redness. He carefully pressed his gloved fingers over the reddened area to assess the character of the tissue for the presence of an abscess. At one point, Dr. Slone paused and explored meticulously the front of his shin. He looked at Mr. Lutz and said, "I think you have an abscess here, sir."

"How did I get an abscess?"

"It's from the infection that started with your injury. Sometimes the infection concentrates in a particular area, and a pocket of pus forms. That's an abscess. I can feel it right here," Dr. Slone said as he pointed to the shin. He continued, "We'll need to drain that with a small incision. We can do it later this morning, if it's okay with you."

"Will it hurt?"

"We'll numb the area with an injection, so you won't feel much. The injection is probably the worst pain," Dr. Slone said, with a reassuring smile.

"Okay. Let's get on with it."

"I'll come back a little later and drain the abscess," said Dr. Slone. He paused and moved from the foot of the bed to Mr. Lutz's side. He continued, "Mr. Lutz, this is a simple problem, and we'll get it taken care of.

"There's another important matter we need to talk about, though. That's what you think about end-of-life issues."

Mr. Lutz glanced at his wife, and his eyes darted back to Dr. Slone. "You think I'm gonna die?"

"No sir, but we need to be prepared. We don't want to do anything that you don't want done."

Mr. Lutz breathed a sigh of relief and said, "I thought maybe this was worse than I thought." He managed to chuckle.

"Your medical problem is simple, and it's also routine for us to talk to our patients about their plans for the end of their lives. Have you thought about that?"

Mr. Lutz perked up. He looked at his wife, nodded, then looked back to Dr. Slone. "Elaine and I took care of all that. We have a Living Will and we've granted our oldest son power of attorney for health care. Our funeral expenses are completely paid, and we have a burial plot at Libertyville Cemetery," he said, as he puffed his chest and winked.

"I'm impressed. Most people don't think ahead like that, but there's another issue we need to address."

"What's that? I thought we had our bases covered."

"We need to discuss Code status." Dr. Slone paused. "Has anyone brought that issue up with you before?"

Mr. Lutz glanced at his wife. She shook her head. Then he said, "I've never heard of Code status, Dr. Slone."

"When you're in the hospital, we do everything to treat illness and keep you alive. Now, like I said, you're in no imminent danger, but we need to know where you stand. If your heart stops while you're here, we would try to restart your heart and bring you back. Did you know that?"

"Heck no," he roared. "I thought the Living Will covered that. Elaine and I don't want anything like that done to us. I don't want to die, but if my heart stops, don't resuscitate me. Let me go."

Mr. Lutz stopped and looked down. He shook his head and said, "Two of my buddies went through that. They got resuscitated and both died...and they both suffered.

"I hated seeing them with all those tubes. They both had a tube in their mouth for breathing and one in their nose for feeding. When they woke up, I could tell they were in pain by their gagging and grimacing. Don't ever put me through that," he said, pointing at Dr. Slone.

"That's why I brought it up, sir. In most cases, the Living Will does not deal with Code status. If your heart or breathing stops, you do not want heroic measures. No machines, no shocks, no chest compressions. Is that right?"

"That's right. Let me die in peace. I want to die naturally." He looked at Elaine, and she nodded in agreement.

"Okay sir, to make this official, we need to complete a form that changes your status to Do Not Resuscitate or DNR. I'll complete my part, and then you'll need to sign it. You will receive a copy, too."

"All right," Mr. Lutz said. Then his face wrinkled, and he lifted a cup to spit. He'd been chewing a tiny plug of tobacco despite his nurse's plea to stop. He sat forward and drew closer to Dr. Slone and asked, "Hey, Doc, what if I would have croaked this morning?"

Dr. Slone sighed deeply and said, "Mr. Lutz, I'm sorry and embarrassed to say that the doctors and nurses would have tried to resuscitate you."

Mr. Lutz's face flushed and he sat up straight. He gritted his teeth. "You better never let that happen."

Dr. Slone stepped back and said, "I'm sorry that no one on our staff asked you about this."

"How in the world does something like this get screwed up?" Mr. Lutz was genuinely curious, as well as angry.

"Did someone ask you if you had a Living Will or an advance directive?"

"Yeah. I told them I had a Living Will. What's an advance directive?"

"An advance directive is any document that communicates your end-of-life wishes. Did they ask you any other questions after you told them you have a Living Will?"

"Nope. I figured it was settled."

"That's the problem. It's a problem in medicine. Not just at this hospital or in this state, but in most states. People derive a false sense of security from a Living Will."

"A false sense of security?"

"That's what you had. You had the sense that you had answered your end-of-life questions through your Living Will, but you didn't.

The Living Will in this state is grossly inadequate for people like you."

"Why's that?" Mr. Lutz's curiosity trumped his anger as he engaged.

"The Living Will specifies one's wishes if they have a terminal illness or they are in a permanently unconscious state, but it does not address Code status. So in a case like yours, the Living Will would not be effective if your heart were to stop. You'd be resuscitated. You must specify, Do Not Resuscitate."

"Oh Lord. That's a truckload of bull. How did we ever get to this point?"

"They wrote the Living Will laws to deal with conditions like comas or terminal illnesses when patients couldn't speak for themselves." Dr. Slone's voice quickened, as his teaching strength emerged. "Remember some of those big lawsuits that argued about whether to keep people alive with machines or with feeding tubes?"

"Oh yeah. I remember that. I wouldn't want that to happen to me."

"Me neither," said Dr. Slone with a smile. He continued, "The Living Will works in situations like those but is inadequate for circumstances like yours. You thought you had all bases covered with your Living Will, but no one talked to you about Code status and resuscitation."

"So what are we gonna do about it?"

"I'm writing the order right now. I need you to sign this form after you read it. We'll make sure the nurses know about the change in Code status, too."

"I don't mean about me," Mr. Lutz said. "I mean what are we gonna do about all the other people who think the same thing I do? You know, all those old folks like me who don't want their chest pumped on and think they have it covered with their Living Will."

Silence filled the room. Dr. Slone's eyes met Mr. Lutz's, and he asked, "What would you do?"

"I'd scrap that Living Will and start over so the document could address Code status. And for now, I'd be sure the attorney or anyone who oversees a Living Will informs people about the shortcomings. They gotta tell people that most Living Wills don't deal with Code status. Then you guys need to get your act together and talk to your patients sooner."

Dr. Slone nodded his head. "You're right. We need to get our act together."

Mr. Lutz spit again and winked at them, as they turned toward the door and left.

Later that day when Kate walked onto the sixth floor, Jack was scanning lab values on the computer. He looked up and turned to Kate. "I did that chart review."

Kate's pulse quickened as she tried to appear uninterested. "Did you find anything interesting?"

"I found that you had reviewed the chart last week."

"Do you have a problem with that?" Kate sounded defensive.

"I just wondered why you rushed down there to see it. The clerk told me you were in."

"I just wanted to go over the case myself and be sure I didn't miss anything."

"Speaking of missing… Do you know anything about missing EKG monitor strips? It looked to me like there should have been some recordings around the time of the Code that were not there."

Kate stood up and glared at Jack. "I don't know what you're talking about. Are you blaming me?"

"Blaming you?" Jack looked bewildered initially, but then his focus returned.

"Blaming you for what?" He turned toward her and sat erect.

Kate collected her wits. "I thought you were blaming me for the chart being messed up."

"You're acting really weird, Simon. What's going on?"

"Nothing's going on, Jack. I'm still sad about the way this case turned out, and I feel responsible for the bad outcome."

"The outcome wasn't that bad until she coded. Do you feel responsible for that?"

Kate was agitated. "She coded because her heart stopped. I didn't have anything to do with that."

"I just wondered why you're so defensive and angry."

"I told you why. I think we should just drop this."

"I'll think about it, Simon." With that, Jack turned and walked away.

Kate's hands were trembling, as she made her way to the call room. She locked herself in a sleeping room and wept.

31

Later that week, Kate was seeing patients with Dr. Dawson and Jack in the ICU. There was a new patient who had an irregular heart rhythm. After examining the patient, Dr. Dawson sat down in front of the computer to look over the abnormalities.

Before he finished, he rolled the mouse to the edge of the screen and inadvertently touched a button that brought up a long list of names.

"Whoops. I've never seen that screen before," Dr. Dawson said. "I don't even know how I got to it."

Kate scanned the list, and she recognized several names. They were patients she'd treated and released from the ICU. She glanced over and could see Jack studying the list, too.

Dr. Dawson clicked on one of the names, and a message popped onto the screen: "Data on this patient has been archived. Please consult with Information Technology (IT) for more information."

Dr. Dawson said, "Archived, huh? I thought they deleted all those old patient files, but I guess not."

He went back to the list and paged down. Kate watched the names flash by—Masterson, O'Brien, Olmstead. Kate's heart stood still. The next name—Pelino. Kate said nothing and tried to pretend that she didn't notice the name. She glanced at Jack to see if he noticed, but she detected no response.

She didn't hear anything else Dr. Dawson said about the patient because she was consumed, thinking how she might erase the files that contained Maria's alarms. Meg could help. She was a genius with computers, but Kate knew that meant she would have to tell Meg everything.

When they finished rounds, Jack gave Kate a long list of work to attend to; longer than usual it seemed. Kate rushed to get it done, so she could get down to IT.

Right after the regular noon case conference, Kate made her way to the IT department, which was tucked away in a hidden corner of the basement. A friendly receptionist greeted her. "May I help you?"

"Yes, please. I'm interested in finding out how I can retrieve some old EKG alarms from the database."

The receptionist laughed and said, "That's a popular question today. One of your colleagues, Dr. Gerard, had the same question and left here with a stack of paper."

Kate felt like someone had hit her in the gut. She closed her eyes and winced.

"Are you all right, Dr. Simon?"

Kate said nothing for several seconds. "I'll be okay. I'm not feeling well today. Could you help me with that alarm question?"

"Come back here to this terminal. The program is still up from Dr. Gerard's research."

Kate looked at the screen. It was Maria Pelino's record. She clicked through the alarms, and the five key records she had deleted from the paper chart were right there in front of her, intact in the electronic record.

She highlighted Maria Pelino's name and pressed "Delete."

The computer beeped and a window appeared: "These files can only be deleted by hospital administration."

She tried again. Another beep. Another window.

Kate stared at the screen for five minutes, logged out, and left the office.

32

"Meg, I need to see you right away."

"What's wrong? Kate, are you okay?"

Meg's voice sounded far away through the cell phone. "I'm fine. Can you meet me in the park across the street from Mercy right away?"

"Sure. I'll be right down."

Thirty minutes later, Kate watched Meg pull in and hurry across the lawn to the picnic table where she sat.

"Kate, you look sick. You're so pale. Hey, you've been crying."

"I've gotten myself into a real bind, Meg." Tears started to roll.

"What happened?"

"I'm so sorry to bring you into this. I hoped that I would never need to tell you and burden you." She stopped and held her head in her hands.

"You know the case that drove me crazy over the past several weeks and the lady finally died a couple weeks ago?"

"How could I forget?"

"I let her die."

"You let her die? What do you mean?"

"She died because I took her off the ventilator."

"You what?!"

"When they decided to release her from Mercy and leave her on life support indefinitely, I let her die naturally. That's what she wanted."

"This is unbelievable. I know that's what she wanted, but what about your life, Kate?"

"I didn't expect to get caught. I really screwed up."

"What happened?"

"I thought I had everything covered, but while we were looking at the computer today, we came across a way to get old electronic records, and hers were still there. Jack saw it, too, and went straight to IT to pull the record. I think it's over."

"How can I help?" Meg looked desperate.

For a moment, Kate thought about asking her sister to hack into the hospital computer records, knowing Meg could probably pull it off. Instead, she started to cry.

"There's nothing you can do, Meg. I just wanted you to know."

Kate clung to Meg and they both wept.

Meg asked, "What do you think will happen?"

"Jack has the evidence and he's always looking for a way to put me down, so things look bad."

"What will you do?"

"I'll tell them that I did what the patient requested and acted in her best interest."

"That sounds good to you and me but what about legally?"

"I'm in big trouble."

Kate's cell phone buzzed. She looked at the text message and sat in silence.

"What was that?"

"That was Jack. He wants to meet in Dr. Dawson's office now."

Kate grabbed Meg's hand. "Meg, I feel like running away, but I'm not very good at that. I've been miserable since she died. I can't keep secrets very well. I need to face the truth and take a stand."

They wept together for several minutes, and then they hugged. Kate made her way slowly across the park toward the hospital with Meg watching until her sister vanished around the corner.

33

When Kate stepped off the elevator, Jack was leaving Dr. Dawson's office. He stopped in his tracks when he saw Kate and waited for her to close the distance.

Kate wanted to turn and run but she walked on. Jack's familiar sneer consumed his face. He shook his head and said, "Well, DoGood, you've got a lot of explaining to do."

Kate kept walking without a word toward Jack and entered Dr. Dawson's office. His receptionist led her to his private office. He looked up from his desk with a bewilderment that Kate had never seen in his eyes.

"Hello, Kate. Close the door and have a seat."

Kate sat on the edge of the chair adjacent his desk.

"Jack's been investigating some inconsistencies in Mrs. Pelino's medical records, and I need to discuss them with you."

"Okay," said Kate softly.

"After we discovered those electronic monitor files this morning, Jack investigated and found some crucial tracings that were missing from the medical record." He pushed two pages toward Kate.

"This one shows Mrs. Pelino's EKG about 20 minutes before she arrested. Then here's an area that looks like artifact followed by a completely different EKG pattern."

These were the same tracings Kate had removed from the chart. She stared at the paper and remained silent.

Dr. Dawson pushed another paper across his desk. "The EKG remained the same with minor variations in rate until suddenly, after another artifact, the EKG went flat-line."

He pulled out another paper. "The tracings of the oxygen saturations are very unusual, too. These important tracings are not in the paper chart, and in fact, we believe someone has tampered with the chart.

"Kate." He waited for her to look up. "Do you know anything about this?"

Kate looked back down. "Maybe the nurse forgot to include those tracings."

"That's possible, but these tracings just don't make sense." He pointed to the EKG tracings. "Look. These are not the same person."

Kate didn't lift her head. She knew the tracings all too well.

"I know you were with Mrs. Pelino when she died, and Jack told me that you reviewed the chart before he did."

"That's all true."

"I called security, and they have contacted the police about this case because we need a careful analysis of the chart to determine if someone altered it."

Kate felt like she'd been slugged in the gut. She sat silently for several seconds. She imagined herself running through the park with Meg, running through the streets of Phnom Penh with her dad, and never coming back.

Dr. Dawson asked, "Kate, can you tell me what happened?"

"I'm sorry, Dr. Dawson." Kate paused. "I couldn't stand seeing Mrs. Pelino leave Mercy. I couldn't let her down."

She watched helplessly as he digested the cascading truth. Kate felt terror as a look of shock and horror spread across Dr. Dawson's face in that instant.

Kate continued, "That EKG tracing for 20 minutes before the arrest is mine and so is the oxygen monitor tracing." She dropped her head. She was too exhausted to cry.

"What did you do?"

"I let Mrs. Pelino die in peace. She was comfortable and died without pain. She was far gone by the time I called the Code. I'm sure she didn't suffer." Kate's voice trailed off.

Dr. Dawson shook his head in disbelief and looked away. His voice broke as he said, "Oh, Kate. What were you thinking?" Kate felt his distress and disappointment.

"I couldn't stand the thought of her going out of here and living on a ventilator, knowing that I caused her pain." She drew a deep breath and waited for Dr. Dawson to look back up. "I didn't plan to get caught. The whole thing seemed foolproof."

Dr. Dawson looked back at Kate. "You know what you've done is unprofessional and illegal. I'm going to have to involve hospital administration and security." Kate sat silently. The weight of her predicament and Dr. Dawson's disappointment crushed her.

Dr. Dawson picked up the phone and called Dr. Zwick. "Jim, we've got a big problem. I need you in my office now." He hung up and sat silently across the desk from Kate.

Dr. Zwick was there within minutes, and Dr. Dawson filled him in on all the details. Dr. Zwick turned to Kate and said, "Dr. Simon, this is a crime. I'm calling hospital security to stay with you until the police arrive."

Kate closed her eyes and dropped her head on the desk.

34

The next three hours were a blur. Detectives read Kate her Miranda rights, then questioned her, cuffed her, and hauled her to jail. Never in her most horrid nightmares could Kate imagine departing Mercy in chains. The squad car thundered past familiar sites, and Kate yearned to run through the park with the wind in her face. Her career in medicine was over; she would never live out her dream. In these few months, Dr. Simon tasted the delight derived from saving a life, and she found what it meant to care deeply for people. That was gone.

The police booked Kate and took a mug shot. More detectives questioned her at the station. Her story was simple: "I helped my patient have what she wanted. Mrs. Pelino wanted to die, and I let her die. I refused to prolong her dying." Kate had nothing to hide, so she disclosed her scheme to dupe the alarms and fulfill her mission of mercy.

Kate was seated in her cell when the guard grunted, "Simon, visitor for you. Come on."

Kate jumped up and followed the guard to a small room. She entered and saw what looked like a row of study cubicles from the med school library. Around the corner, there was a window at the front of each cubicle. She went to the third cubicle. Staring through the glass was Meg. The sisters threw their arms toward each other and stopped.

Meg wept at the sight of Kate's bloodshot eyes and wrinkled gray prison uniform. The agony Kate saw in Meg's face broke her heart, knowing that she was the author of Meg's misery. Both were overwhelmed by their uncertain future. Both sobbed with hands pressed against the glass.

Finally Kate said, "Meg, I'm so scared. I'm sorry I got you into this."

Meg gazed through the scratched Plexiglas and saw exhaustion and fear consuming her sister. Meg nudged forward and asked, "Wasn't there any other way?"

Kate thought for a few seconds, shook her head, and said, "No. Her son planned to transfer her to the other hospital, and she could have lingered there for months. I couldn't let him prolong her dying." She hesitated then added, "She just wanted to die naturally."

Meg dropped her chin and shook her head ever so slightly. "Why did you sacrifice so much? She was old and wouldn't have lived long. You have your entire future."

"I thought about my future. That woman told me she didn't want any of that heroic medical care. I betrayed her. I couldn't live with myself. Besides, I didn't plan to be caught."

"Why didn't you tell me what you were thinking? I remember how weird you were acting that day before she died."

"I didn't want to drag you into this."

"But Kate, look what's happened now."

"I think I did the right thing. She told me what she wanted, and I carried out her will when she couldn't."

"But Kate, that's a crime."

Kate's expression hardened. "I know that's the letter of the law, but I think we can beat these charges. I did exactly what Maria wanted and I'll prove it."

Meg shook her head. "You are a stubborn woman."

"We'll show everyone that her son is the villain, not me."

"Okay, Kate, let's do it. My boss is well connected, and he can help us find a good attorney."

"Thanks, Meg."

Meg looked down, collecting her thoughts. "Dr. Dawson called me today, Kate. Since he'll have to testify for the prosecution, the DA insisted he not see you before or during the trial."

Tears welled in Kate's eyes. She felt like she had lost her father a second time. She knew that her actions would lead to more problems for Dr. Dawson since he was in charge and ultimately responsible for Mrs. Pelino's case. Finally Kate said, "I feel so bad about how this is going to affect Dr. Dawson."

Just then their privacy vanished as the door creaked and the guard shouted, "Time's up, Simon."

Uncertainty and disappointment flooded their eyes as they said goodbye. Both wondered when, or if, Kate would get her life back.

35

Kate was indicted for aggravated murder since she had planned and deliberately ended Mrs. Pelino's life. TV crews surrounded the courthouse and hospital. Kate's mug shot and story made front-page news nationwide.

Headlines included, "Reckless Intern Pulls Plug," "Cold-Blooded Murder in the ICU," and "Helpless Woman Dies with Murderer at Bedside." Dr. Jack Gerard was the hero.

The *Herald* read as follows:

A Mercy Medical Center intern disconnected a critically ill, 83-year-old woman from life support against her son's wishes, resulting in the woman's death two weeks ago.

Dr. Kate Simon, 27, was taken into custody and charged with aggravated murder. She was in her third month of training at Mercy when she removed life support care from Maria Pelino, who was in critical condition after suffering a stroke.

Pelino died within 20 minutes of being disconnected from her respirator, according to a Mercy spokesperson. She was scheduled to be transferred from Mercy later that day, according to hospital officials.

The alleged murder was discovered by Dr. Jack Gerard, a third-year resident, who had been tasked with investigating Pelino's death.

"Simon tried to cover her tracks by altering several of the physical records taken at the time of Pelino's death," said Gerard. "But she either was unaware of the existence of electronic records archived in Mercy's IT department, or was unable to change them.

"The electronic records told me everything I needed to know about how Maria Pelino died, and how Simon carried it out."

One of her fellow interns visited Kate at the jail and told her Jack was basking in the limelight. He boasted about his interviews and recorded every news story and made a DVD. At Mercy, the intern heard Jack say, "Dr. DoGood turned out to be bad after all."

The judge held Kate without bail since she faced a potential life sentence.

Time went so slowly in jail. Kate spent hour after hour rehashing her decision. Each time she came to the same conclusion: I could not prolong her dying.

In her selfish moments, she wished Dr. Dawson had never raised the issue of Code status and resuscitation.

Then she would scold herself. "This is not about me. This is about Mrs. Pelino." She hoped someone would embrace her side of the story.

Meg, with the help of her boss, acquired an experienced attorney for Kate, and they began to prepare. Paul Bence was 57 and had fiery blue eyes. He kept fit physically and mentally. He had experience in criminal law and malpractice defense, so he understood the medical community and could work with doctors.

From the beginning, Paul told Kate that the cards were stacked against her. With her confession and all the evidence, it would be impossible to raise doubt in any juror's mind about her guilt.

Paul had been in conversation with the DA who offered to plea bargain. They would accept a guilty plea to murder. With that, Kate could expect 15 years to life. The DA promised to recommend the minimal sentence.

Paul warned Kate that if her case went to trial and she were convicted of aggravated murder she would receive a mandatory life sentence.

"I'm not interested in the plea deal," Kate said with quiet determination.

Paul's words were stern and precise. "Do you understand that an aggravated murder conviction will lead to a mandatory life sentence?"

"I understand. Mr. Bence, I'm not really sure you understand me." Kate tried hard not to be rude, but she was annoyed. "I did not kill Mrs. Pelino. I let her die.

"She was at the end of her life, and she wanted to die. She told me that as plainly as you said 'mandatory life sentence.'" Kate jumped up and blasted the table with her fist. "My crime was my failure to document my conversation and have her sign my note."

"So, that's a 'no' on the plea bargain?" Paul asked, as he lifted an eyebrow.

Kate nodded and said, "Mr. Bence, I did the right thing. What I need you to do is help me prove that I did the right thing." She stared into his eyes and wondered if Paul was the man for the job.

He hesitated for a few seconds. Then he looked her in the eye and extended his right hand. "I'm ready to defend you. Are you ready to get to work, Dr. Simon?"

Kate's face softened. "Thanks, Mr. Bence. Work sounds awesome. I'm so bored in here." Kate wiped her eye as she forced a smile.

"Call me Paul. We have a lot of thinking and planning ahead of us." With that, his inquiry began, and they built their case against daunting odds. They would have to convince a jury that Kate did the right thing by refusing to prolong Maria Pelino's dying.

Over the next several weeks, Paul developed a growing vigor for the case and the cause. He began to see the issues with mounting clarity. One day when he came to meet with Kate, he could hardly contain himself.

"I can't believe how many families have gone through terrible experiences with loved ones at the end of life. I spoke with two friends this week with similar stories. They both had elderly parents who died after weeks of care that didn't help them. It only prolonged their dying. Just like your patient, Mrs. Pelino."

Paul continued, "You also got me thinking about my own family. I have an uncle whose health is failing. He still thinks clearly, but he needs to go into a nursing home because he can't take care of himself. I took care of his will and his Living Will, but I had not discussed Code status with him until now.

"He was so relieved to let us know what he wanted done. He clearly does not want resuscitation and life support, and now we know. I asked his doctor to complete the DNR forms, and we have them on file now."

Kate smiled, realizing that at least some good had come from her disaster.

Paul's excitement persisted. "I went to the senior center Mrs. Pelino frequented and talked to the Knit-Wits. Remember you told me about the knitting club?"

Kate nodded. "Sure."

"One of those ladies, Francis McMillan, is a real fireball. She's sharp, witty, and can recount Mrs. Pelino's story vividly. She remembers Maria telling her and the members of the group that she would not want prolonged life support. She's agreed to testify."

"That's fantastic." Paul's enthusiasm renewed Kate's spirits and helped her concentrate on the arduous preparation.

The day before Kate's trial, they worked hard for several hours. As their meeting wound down, Kate asked, "How long do you think this will take?"

"It shouldn't take more than a few days. Their case against you is simple. Her son, the next of kin, wanted her alive, and you killed her," Paul said without hesitation or emotion. He saw Kate swallow hard and look down.

He moved toward her, gripped her shoulder, and with firmness said, "I don't think you killed her, Kate. You did the right thing. That's our case. It's simple, too. You granted her wish and refused to prolong her dying."

Sleep didn't come easy that night. Kate kept wondering whether any juror would understand her actions.

36

When Kate entered the courtroom, her eyes met those of Meg, who sat in the first row. She saw Dr. Dawson seated a few rows back and longed to sit down and talk with him. Everyone stood as Judge Anthony Perry entered the courtroom. He was near retirement but remained astute, and Paul was glad to have him presiding.

Kate didn't know what to think of the courtroom scene. It was all foreign to her. She felt odd sitting at a desk in a navy blue business suit after three months in the drab jail outfit.

The crammed courtroom astonished Kate, and she noticed press passes throughout. She had almost forgotten the headlines and all the interest.

She scanned the crowd and stopped, as she met familiar eyes. Her blood went cold and her gut was hollow, as the memorable sneer spread across his face. Dr. Gerard had come to settle the score. Kate looked down and turned away.

After a few formalities, jury selection commenced and lasted all day. Judge Perry adjourned until the next morning. Then the war began. The District Attorney, a bright and striking woman with years of experience, engaged the battle in her opening statement. She had tried numerous murderers, but this case was distinct. She would never get a case like this again.

Her opening statement was clear and concise. She summarized the case crisply. "We will show that Dr. Simon took Mrs. Pelino's life into her hands and ended it."

The DA lingered over those words for a few seconds then turned toward the jury.

"Dr. Simon believed she was acting on behalf of Mrs. Pelino, but overstepped her authority and the law. She planned Mrs. Pelino's death and carried her plan out precisely. Mrs. Pelino was murdered in her hospital bed with Dr. Simon, her physician and killer, at her bedside."

She continued, "Our case is straightforward and unambiguous. First, we will show that Mr. Pelino, the victim's next of kin, explicitly and repeatedly stated his desire that his mother be kept alive.

"Then we will show that Dr. Simon planned and caused Mrs. Pelino's death. Dr. Simon sat at her bedside and watched her take her last breaths, when she had the power to prolong her life.

"Her crime is premeditated murder, and the charge is aggravated murder. As a society, we cannot allow a physician or any health care provider to take a life into her own hands like Dr. Simon has done."

The DA took her seat and Paul stood. "Your Honor, I request permission to present my opening statement after the prosecution has called her witnesses."

Judge Perry glanced at the DA and said, "Permission granted."

The DA stood and said, "I would like to call our first witness, Mr. Thomas Pelino."

He climbed to the stand, and the bailiff swore him in. The DA succinctly established Mr. Pelino as the next of kin and Mrs. Pelino's only heir. She moved then to the crux of the issue.

"As next of kin, did you understand that you were your mother's medical decision maker?"

"Yes. There are no other relatives."

"What decisions did you make on your mother's behalf?"

"I had to decide whether or not my mother would receive the care she needed. They asked me about various medical procedures and most of all, whether to let my mother live or die."

"Please summarize your decisions."

"I wanted everything done. I wanted them to do everything in their power to keep her alive and make her better."

"Who were your mother's doctors?"

"Dr. Dawson was the main doctor. Doctor..." He paused and with a scowl he snapped, "I hate to use that term for her, but Dr. Simon was the other one."

"How would you describe your relationship with these doctors?"

"Tense. I felt pressured by both doctors to let my mother die. They wanted me to consent to a DNR status. You know, Do Not Resuscitate. They brought the issue up about every day. I finally asked them to quit harassing me about it," grunted Mr. Pelino.

"When did the DNR issue first surface?"

"Dr. Simon asked me about Code status in our first phone conversation. That's when she told me about the stroke and my mother's condition. I thought it was inappropriate then and I still do. I couldn't believe that she was bringing up Code status while I was in shock, hearing about my mother's illness for the first time."

"What made the Code status question inappropriate?"

"I had so much to think about. In one sentence, she told me Mother had a major stroke and might die. In the next sentence, she wanted to know if they could let her die. I still can't believe she treated me that way."

"When did the issue come up again?"

"As soon as I arrived at Mercy, Dr. Simon and Dr. Dawson attacked me with questions about Code status. For three or four days, it came up daily. They finally backed off when I told them to quit harassing me. I told them to do everything to help Mother."

He stopped for a few seconds; then with a quickening pace and escalating tone he thundered, "Every time there was a change in my mother's condition or she needed a procedure, they would go right back to the DNR question. It was relentless." He breathed rapidly as his eyes darted between Dr. Dawson and Kate.

"Was Dr. Simon involved in the conversations about the DNR status?"

"Of course," he barked. "Dr. Simon knew what I wanted, and she killed my mother."

The DA paused to let the words descend on the jury. Then she said, "To summarize, first, you are the next of kin and have the legal right to make decisions for your mother. Second, you requested the doctors to do everything to sustain your mother's life. Third, Dr. Simon was part of these conversations and unmistakably understood your wishes. And last, you felt pressured to withdraw care by Dr. Simon. Is that right?"

"Yes, it is."

"No more questions," she said, as she circled past the jury.

Paul stood and walked toward Mr. Pelino. He looked him in the eye and asked, "How well would you say you knew your mother?"

"I knew her all my life and knew her well."

"When was the last time you talked to your mother?"

"About 10 years ago." Mr. Pelino said it as if all people visited their mother once a decade.

"Ten years." Paul lifted an eyebrow and with a touch of sarcasm added, "That's a long time between visits. What happened?"

"After my father's death, we had a disagreement. We never reconciled. I guess we both got busy." He shrugged his shoulders. His voice remained casual and his face expressionless, but he began to shift in his chair and his foot began to tap.

"Did you ever try to contact your mother?"

Kate watched his jaw muscle start to twitch. His eyes remained fixed. "No," he said.

"Did she ever try to contact you?"

"No." His jaw twitched again.

"So, Mr. Pelino, you abandoned your mother in her later years because of a spat over money. You were overcome with guilt when she became ill and wanted to be her hero."

"Objection, Your Honor! Counsel is badgering the witness," shouted the DA.

"Sustained. Mr. Bence, redirect your questions," said Judge Perry.

Paul took a deep breath and proceeded, "Did you feel guilty for not having contact with your elderly mother for 10 years?"

"Not really." He worked hard to resume an air of nonchalance.

Paul matched Mr. Pelino's indifference with disbelief. "So you were content to avoid your mother for 10 years? No big deal?" Paul's brow furrowed with doubt.

"I wasn't happy. I wanted it to be different." His feigned indifference began to disintegrate, and his face hardened.

"Did you want your mother to recover, so you could speak to her again?"

"Yes," he said in a tone that could barely be heard. His jaw was clenched again. Sweat beaded on his forehead. He brushed it away with a swift swipe.

"What chance of recovery did Dr. Dawson tell you she had?"

"He told me she probably wouldn't be able to talk."

"What chance of recovery to normal life did they tell you she had?"

"They said she wouldn't recover. They said she probably wouldn't walk again."

"What did they recommend?"

Mr. Pelino's face stiffened, and he leaned forward on the rail. "They wanted me to agree to withdraw life support. I told you that already!"

"Why did you reject their advice?"

"I knew my mother, and I knew she was a fighter. I knew she could make it."

"Did you believe the doctors were against you?"

"Yes. They wanted to let her die from the beginning," he snarled.

"In your opinion, you acted in your mother's best interest against the doctors who did not want what was best for her. Is that right?"

"Yes, it was me against them. Dr. Dawson and Dr. Simon were always talking about DNR and Comfort Care. I got so sick of it. I just wanted my mother to be able to talk to me again." His voice trailed off, and the jury fixed their eyes on him.

Paul sensed the jury's concern. He paused to allow Mr. Pelino to collect himself. Then he asked, "Did you ever speak to your mother about death?"

"My mother was full of life. She was always active and into all kinds of things..." said Mr. Pelino.

Paul interrupted, "Mr. Pelino, I asked if you ever discussed death with your mother. I'll repeat the question: Did you ever discuss death with your mother?"

Mr. Pelino's face softened; he dropped his head and said, "No."

"So you don't know how she felt about death in general, and specifically about her own death. Is that correct, sir?" Paul's energy grew.

With his chin down and voice faint, he said, "Yes."

"Did Dr. Simon tell you that she discussed death with your mother?"

His anger returned. "She harassed me several times," he roared. The flow of sweat resumed.

"Would you please recount what Dr. Simon told you?"

"Dr. Simon said my mother told her she did not want life-saving measures."

"And what was your response?"

"I didn't believe it!" shouted Mr. Pelino.

"Why not?"

"I told you, my mother loved life too much." His facial twitch reappeared.

"But you said death was never a topic of discussion, correct?"

Mr. Pelino shifted uncomfortably. "I told you that, too. I knew my mother!"

"But you didn't speak to her for 10 years. People change in 10 years. Do you think it's possible that your mother did not want life-saving care?"

Mr. Pelino sat in silence for several seconds while he glared at Paul. Then, looking directly at Kate, he shouted, "Impossible!"

"No more questions." Paul marched back toward Kate.

Next the prosecution's star witness stepped forward. Dr. Jack Gerard wore a new tailored suit that would look good on the evening news. Kate thought he looked like he'd visited the dentist to whiten his teeth.

"Obnoxious as ever," she muttered under her breath.

Jack demonstrated confidence and competence as he answered the DA's questions. Kate could tell he enjoyed being the detective who unraveled her scheme. He spoke in animated detail about his growing suspicions toward Dr. Simon and how he discovered the computer records. Finally he spoke about his skepticism regarding the integrity of the paper chart. He said he was sure someone had tampered with it.

The DA introduced printed records of the EKG and oxygen-monitoring data. Jack explained the findings with precision and clarity. The DA was impressed. The jury was impressed. The crowd was impressed. And of course, Jack appeared impressed. The DA portrayed him as the hero and protector of humanity.

She concluded her questions with, "Thank you for your testimony, Dr. Gerard. We are fortunate to have physicians like you who are committed to looking out for our good." Several jurors nodded. Kate shuddered. Jack smiled and glanced her way.

Paul's next move floored Kate. He stood and said, "No questions at this time, but Your Honor, I reserve the right to recall this witness." Paul gave Kate a wink as he returned to his seat, and she breathed a sigh of relief.

Kate saw the arrogant confidence swell in Jack. She could tell he thought even the defense attorney respected and feared him. He tightened his bright blue tie and swaggered to his seat. Kate figured he was getting ready for another afternoon of TV interviews.

Next the DA called Dr. Dawson and two detectives to recount Dr. Simon's confession, attempting to prove that Kate planned the murder. It was all clear. Then the DA presented more evidence to supplement the confession, including fingerprints from the chart with microscopic evidence implicating Kate as the one who had tampered with the chart.

The evidence was irrefutable. Everything fit. Kate planned it and did it. Paul was powerless in the face of such obvious proof. The DA concluded her case, and Judge Perry adjourned court for the day.

Paul hoped the jurors would be able to see the evidence in a different light when court came to order the next day.

37

The crowd rose as Judge Perry entered. Kate noticed Jack's smirk as he caught her eyes. She knew he loved the spotlight and wouldn't miss this spectacle for anything.

Paul took the floor and went to work. He summarized the defense case saying, "The state has demonstrated that Dr. Simon helped Mrs. Pelino die. We do not dispute that claim. We will show that Dr. Simon acted according to Mrs. Pelino's wishes.

"Mrs. Pelino did not want to live dependent on machines and medicines. She did not want anyone to prolong her dying." Paul paused to let those three words settle and then continued, "Therefore, Dr. Simon acted in Mrs. Pelino's best interest. She did this at great personal risk. Her motive was compassion, not malice. Her action was not murder; it was mercy."

Paul paused and turned toward the judge. He said, "Your Honor, our first witness is the defendant, Dr. Kate Simon."

Kate's mouth was dry and her stomach growled. She didn't eat that morning. She took a sip of water, stood up slowly, and tried to walk with confidence.

Paul first established Kate's role as an intern at Mercy and then asked, "Dr. Simon, when and where did you meet Mrs. Pelino?"

"I met her on August 20 in the clinic at Mercy."

"What transpired during your meeting?"

"I performed a complete history and physical."

"What did you find?"

"I found her to be an active elderly woman who took care of herself. The only abnormality I found was a carotid bruit."

"Please explain what that is and its significance, Dr. Simon."

"A bruit is a blowing sound heard with a stethoscope over an artery. It usually indicates some blockage of blood flow. Hers was in the carotid artery, which supplies blood to the brain. It is an important finding because it could present a risk for stroke."

"Please explain a stroke."

"A stroke occurs when part of the brain doesn't receive adequate blood flow. A clot can form in an abnormal carotid artery and then break loose and block blood flow to part of the brain. That causes a stroke if it persists."

"Please describe what you and Mrs. Pelino discussed."

"I told her about the bruit and the risk of stroke. I told her that we needed to investigate it with a test."

"And how did she respond?"

"She had no interest in testing. I repeated the case for investigation and treatment to reduce stroke risk, and she steadfastly refused. I encouraged her to get the bruit evaluated. She told me that another physician found the bruit earlier, and she refused evaluation at that time, too."

"How did you proceed?"

"She was of sound mind and refused the evaluation, so I didn't pursue it. Every competent patient has the right to decline medical care."

"What did you discuss next?"

"I initiated a conversation about end-of-life decisions. I described what the usual course of resuscitation was like and asked her if she wanted to be resuscitated or maintained on mechanical life support.

"She emphatically told me that she wanted no artificial life support. She told me that she had lived a good life and would not want to live if her quality of life was poor. She wanted to remain active and told me that she would not want to live in an impaired or debilitated state."

Paul turned toward his desk and lifted a medical chart in the air. "Your Honor, I want to introduce this evidence. This is Mrs. Pelino's medical record while under the care of Dr. Miguel Hernandez, who treated Mrs. Pelino before Dr. Simon.

"It clearly documents that Mrs. Pelino declined evaluation of the carotid abnormality a year prior to her visit with Dr. Simon. This demonstrates that she declined health care."

Judge Perry nodded and said, "The exhibit is admitted."

Next Paul lifted a few pages copied from the schedule book at the clinic. He pointed to a few lines and said, "Your Honor, this is the next piece of evidence I wish to present. It is the Mercy Clinic schedule for August 20, and it shows that Mrs. Pelino saw Dr. Simon."

Then Paul turned to Kate and said, "Dr. Simon, there were no records of your visit with Mrs. Pelino. Please explain what happened."

Kate took a deep breath and began deliberately, "After I finished my visit with Mrs. Pelino and before I wrote my note, a

Code Blue was called in the hospital. It was late in the day, and I was on call that night, so I had to respond. I ran out of the clinic.

"Then I got busy and forgot to document my conversation with Mrs. Pelino. I planned to write everything down, and I also planned to have her sign the note to prove her intentions."

Paul returned to the desk and produced another page. He turned toward Judge Perry and said, "Your Honor, this piece of evidence is a log of Code Blue calls at Mercy. You will find that on August 20 at 5:34 p.m. a Code was called, corroborating Dr. Simon's account."

Paul turned back to Kate. "When did you realize your error?"

"Not until it was too late. Mrs. Pelino had a stroke and was in the hospital. She could not speak and therefore could not affirm our discussion. I tried to help Mr. Pelino understand, but he didn't believe me."

"Thanks, Dr. Simon. I will end there for now," said Paul, as he turned away.

The DA rose and headed toward Kate. She watched the DA as if in slow motion. Her deliberate steps prolonged Kate's agony and increased anticipation in the court. She stood before Kate for several seconds and finally began, "How long had you been a doctor when you saw Mrs. Pelino?"

"Two months." It took all her effort to look the DA in the eye and not waver. The jury couldn't see, but her legs shook and she fought off nausea. Kate didn't look down and sat erect.

"How long had you worked in the clinic before you saw Mrs. Pelino?"

"It was my first month in the clinic." Her eyes remained fixed on the DA.

"How many days had you worked in the clinic?"

"It was my first day." Kate knew where the DA was headed and bit the inside of her cheek, trying to keep her composure.

The DA walked slowly away from Kate and said, "When you saw Mrs. Pelino, you had been a doctor for about two months." She stopped, turned on her heel, and stared at Kate. "You claim that Mrs. Pelino refused medical care. How many patients have you cared for who made that decision?"

Kate did not answer immediately. She looked to the side and folded her hands as she thought. "I've helped take care of several patients who refused care."

The DA raised an eyebrow and asked, "Several? Please be more specific."

Kate fended off a wavering voice. "While at Mercy, there have been around 10 or 12, and at least that many as a med student."

"And you believe you're experienced enough to communicate with an elderly patient about her refusal of medical care?"

"I have a lot to learn, but I've had a good teacher. Dr. Dawson repeatedly instructed us about this issue. I watched him talk to several patients in similar circumstances. He trained me well. I knew how to talk to Mrs. Pelino, and I understood her."

Kate could feel her defensiveness welling up. She hated being insulted by this DA, who seemed to know very little about medicine.

The DA stood directly in front of Kate. She crossed her arms, placed her weight on one leg so her hips shifted, and she asked, "Are you certain that Mrs. Pelino did not want life-sustaining care?"

"Certain!" Kate said with more force and volume, as she leaned forward in the chair.

"Is your certainty what prevented you from discussing her case with one of your attendings?" The DA did not take her eyes off Kate. She didn't let Kate answer. "Were you so certain that you didn't need to document your visit with Mrs. Pelino?"

Kate looked to the side and swallowed hard. Her mouth was dry. "Those were both mistakes."

The DA's confidence grew. She turned away from Kate, tossed her head and her long, dark hair followed. "A mistake of inexperience. How can you be so confident about your abilities and perceptions? So confident that you end a patient's life? Young lady, you overestimate yourself."

Paul shot to his feet. "Your Honor, I object," he shouted. "The DA is drawing a conclusion and not asking a question."

Judge Perry turned to the DA. "Sustained."

The DA was still happy. She made her point. Now she turned toward Kate, and in a softer voice with a hint of a smile, she asked, "Do you think you're experienced enough as a physician to have an end-of-life discussion and dictate life and death?"

Kate sat upright, gently lifted her head, and said, "Yes."

With her arms crossed, the DA fixed her eyes on Kate for several seconds to underscore her dissension. She was done for now. She spun toward the judge on one foot. "No more questions, Your Honor." Her eyes darted through the jurors with a contented glance.

Kate looked down for a few seconds as her confidence ebbed. She remembered her conversation with Maria and thought, "Don't give up. You did the right thing." Her chin slowly lifted and her eyes glistened. Kate was not done. She stood with a refreshed air of confidence and strolled back to her seat.

Kate saw a look of relief spread across Meg's face as Meg sensed Kate's confidence returning. This trial was far from over.

38

Dr. Dawson headed to the stand next, and Paul began, "How long have you been in medical practice?"

"About 28 years."

"Please describe your current practice."

"I care for hospitalized patients with medical problems. Our patients come through the emergency department, and if they are sick enough to need admission, I care for them with the residents."

"How many new patients do you see each week?"

"Approximately 20-35 new patients."

"How many are elderly patients?"

"The majority. I don't know exactly. Every year the mean age in the U.S. increases, so we see more elderly patients all the time."

"Do some patients decline health care?"

"Yes."

"Please explain the rationale."

"There are a couple of reasons. All health care comes with a risk/benefit ratio. The risks might outweigh the benefits. For example, a heart-valve surgery in an elderly patient with a weak heart is very risky. It might make more sense to live with the bad valve and decline the surgery.

"Another reason people decline health care is personal preference. Many people reach a stage in their lives where they decide they would rather live more naturally. That is, they would rather not have medical tests and procedures to prolong their lives."

Paul waited a moment before continuing. "You said, 'They would rather live more naturally.' Please elaborate."

"With age, most people develop an expanding list of medical problems. Some problems are easily treatable while others aren't and even progress. Most medical problems are treated with medications or procedures, which typically have some adverse effects.

"Therefore, people find themselves dealing with the problems of aging and the perils of the treatments. Some people decline medical treatments that would potentially prolong their lives, and instead seek out measures that provide comfort."

Paul's eyebrows lifted with his voice. "Why would someone decide against treatment that would prolong life? You imply that some people would rather die." ⎯⎯

Dr. Dawson shifted in his chair. "There comes a point in many people's lives when their quality of life declines and they no longer enjoy life. A person who no longer enjoys quality life may decide against medical treatment.

"Some people prefer to die naturally rather than live on with a poor quality of life. If someone decides to prolong their life in the face of poor quality of life, I believe they are prolonging their dying. They have no long-term benefit from the medical care, and in many cases, they suffer needlessly."

"Do you advise patients on these issues?"

"Certainly. This is an important service I provide to my patients. Most patients and their families do not understand how the medical system works and do not realize that they have the right and privilege to decline health care. Many are relieved to refuse further testing, change the goals of treatment, and focus on Comfort Care."

Paul asked, "Do you believe Dr. Simon was out of line when she raised end-of-life issues with Mr. Pelino during their first conversation?"

"She did exactly what I asked her to do. In fact, I would have reprimanded her if she had neglected the issue."

"Why the urgency?"

"We honor our patient's requests, and we wanted to abide by Mrs. Pelino's wishes."

"Why didn't you stop care as per her requests?"

"We did not have legal documentation of Mrs. Pelino's wishes, so our next step was to rely on her next of kin as her decision maker."

"And what was his decision?"

"Mr. Pelino asked that we provide every possible medical therapy to prolong his mother's life."

"What was your response?"

"I followed his request."

"Mr. Pelino stated that you 'harassed' him about the issue of Code status. Would you describe your interactions with him?"

Dr. Dawson shifted in his chair. "From the beginning, our relationship was adversarial. Mr. Pelino was suspicious of our team because we advocated for what we believed were Mrs. Pelino's wishes. She stated plainly that she did not want artificial life support, and we wanted to comply with those wishes.

"We found ourselves in a difficult position, and we reminded Mr. Pelino of his mother's request at several junctures. I did not harass him."

"What made this situation difficult for you?"

"Mrs. Pelino did not want artificial life support, and we used extraordinary measures to keep her alive. Every day I felt uneasy about the discomfort that she experienced. We prolonged her dying, but we could not provide quality of life."

"Were there any other measures that might have improved her quality of life?"

"Absolutely not. She was near the end of her life, and we were prolonging her dying against her wishes."

"What options did you present to Mr. Pelino?"

"I tried to help him understand the issue of Code status. We resuscitate all patients whose heart or breathing stops unless they decide against resuscitation in advance. Mrs. Pelino did not want resuscitation, so we encouraged Mr. Pelino to opt for Do Not Resuscitate status, DNR. Patients who opt for DNR with Comfort Care receive pain medication and other treatments to keep them comfortable."

"What did he decide?"

"He refused to agree with a DNR status and asked that we do everything for his mother."

"What happened next in her hospital course?"

"She developed pneumonia and needed the support of a ventilator to keep her alive."

"Please describe a ventilator."

"The ventilator is a sophisticated air compressor that pushes air into the lungs. It provides the power, air pressures, and oxygen levels that ill patients need. The air flows through a plastic hose that rests in the mouth and trachea. We tape the tube to the face to hold it in place."

"Describe life on a ventilator."

"It is quite uncomfortable. The plastic tube is six to eight millimeters in diameter and causes gagging. Patients cannot talk with the tube in place. They can't clear their airways with a cough, so we suction the airway with a small plastic tube and that causes discomfort, too.

"They cannot get out of bed, so the immobility produces more discomfort in muscles and joints, as well as pressure changes in the skin. Imagine how you'd feel lying in bed for several days or even weeks. Most patients are heavily sedated, so they can tolerate life on a ventilator."

"What other procedures did Mrs. Pelino require?"

"She needed a tracheostomy tube and a feeding tube. The tracheostomy tube replaces the plastic breathing tube.

"Over time, the plastic tube through the mouth injures the tissues and must be replaced with a tube that's inserted surgically directly into the airway beneath the voice box. The surgeon creates a hole in the airway and inserts the tube. The feeding tube is placed surgically through the abdominal wall into the stomach."

"How does a patient live long-term on a ventilator?"

"The machine breathes for them, and health care workers care for them. They are totally dependent on machines and other people. Most require sedatives and pain medications to tolerate existence. Communication is often very difficult because they cannot speak."

"Did you believe she would recover?"

"No."

"Did you inform Mr. Pelino?"

"Yes."

"And his response?"

"'Do everything to keep my mother alive.'"

"Were you comfortable with that course?"

"No."

"Why?"

"We kept her alive, but we couldn't make her well." Dr. Dawson stopped and shook his head. "She suffered and I suffered watching her. Dr. Simon agonized every day over Mrs. Pelino's misery."

The room was silent. The sound of her own breathing penetrated Kate's ears. Every eye fixed on Dr. Dawson as many in the courtroom seemed to understand, for the first time, the tortures of prolonged dying.

Paul waited for several seconds to let the jolt of truth land squarely.

"Dr. Dawson, I would like to back up now. We need to clarify what is meant by Code status. Please explain Code status."

"In the hospital, if someone's heart or breathing stops, we call a 'Code.' At Mercy, we call it Code Blue. We have a team of professionals that respond to the Code Blue call and make every effort to resuscitate the patient. Unless otherwise specified, every patient's Code status is Full Code, so we call Code Blue if they need resuscitation.

"If someone designates Do Not Resuscitate or DNR, then we note that prominently in the chart, and they wear a special bracelet to mark their status. If their heart or breathing stops, then we do not call a Code Blue."

"Do patients have other choices?"

"Yes. They can choose DNR with Comfort Care only. In that case, they would not receive any medical treatments except to provide comfort. The other option is what we designate DNR with medical interventions. In these cases, patients receive medical and surgical treatments but not resuscitation."

"Give me an example of both."

"DNR Comfort Care only is common in patients with known terminal conditions who are in the late stages of their disease. Many people who know their life is measured in weeks or months decide that they would not want life-prolonging medical treatments. With DNR Comfort Care, if a patient contracts pneumonia, for example, then we do not treat it unless we believe treatment would alleviate suffering. Instead we allow it to run its course, and it could cause death. We keep them comfortable and allow a natural death."

"What about DNR with medical interventions?"

"In that setting, we provide Comfort Care, and we treat other conditions as they arise. Last week I took care of a 90-year-old man who came to the hospital with a fever and back pain. He had a potentially fatal bacterial infection in his kidney. We discussed his situation, and he decided that he wanted us to treat his infection, but he did not want CPR and resuscitation if his heart stopped. Therefore, his status was DNR with medical interventions."

"Did you regard that as a good decision?"

"Yes."

"Please tell me why."

"He was alert and active. He was still able to do many things that he liked, and treatment of the infection was simple. We did not have to subject him to painful procedures or risky medications, so the likelihood of successful treatment that would add quality to his life was very high. That's why medical interventions made sense."

Dr. Dawson paused and then continued. "The DNR decision was a good one, too. At age 90, this patient's chance of surviving resuscitation and being discharged from the hospital is only about five percent." He paused again.

"That means that his chances of a painful resuscitation attempt with prolonged futile care, if he survived a resuscitation attempt, are about 95 percent. That's why I believe he made a good decision to choose DNR."

Paul asked, "What about long-term survival after resuscitation?"

"As you'd expect, survival drops off pretty abruptly because these patients are usually quite ill. One study of in-hospital resuscitations showed 35 percent were initially resuscitated, 12 percent left the hospital, and only eight percent survived six weeks. So, almost a third of their patients who survived to discharge, died within the first six weeks.

"Another study found that 15 percent of resuscitated patients survived to discharge, but only five percent lived for a year. Therefore, only one in three survivors to discharge survived for a year."

"Have most patients talked to their doctors about these facts and their Code status?"

"No, in fact, very few people understand Code status. The sad reality is that many people suffer needlessly and receive medications and procedures they would decline if they understood these facts and their options." Dr. Dawson's words were the same that Kate had heard several times on rounds at Mercy.

His zeal for compassionate treatment of patients flowed forth during his testimony. Kate sensed that everyone could hear and feel his sincerity, and any notion of Dr. Dawson as a "harasser" was put to rest. Kate couldn't help but think about how much she wished she was back on rounds with Dr. Dawson and not seated here as a criminal.

Paul continued. "Why do you think this conversation is not happening?"

"It's a complicated issue, but Dr. Simon's dilemma sheds light on it. One problem is the reluctance on the part of the patient or the family members to discuss the issue. Sometimes people feel like the doctor is giving up on the patient if he or she asks about Code status. Therefore, some doctors are reluctant to address it.

"Besides that, it's a difficult conversation. Most people don't like to discuss death, so initiating the conversation is a taxing job.

"Finally, if we want to talk about real-world limitations, look at the economics. The payment a physician receives for the time and effort that it takes to pull the family and patient together for this important conversation is grossly deficient."

"What was the problem in Mrs. Pelino's case?"

"Dr. Simon acted in good faith. She took time to have the difficult conversation, but she failed to document Mrs. Pelino's desires. Then we were forced to provide unnecessary and unwanted care because Mr. Pelino did not believe Dr. Simon."

"What would have happened if Mr. Pelino would have agreed to Comfort Care according to his mother's stated desire?"

"Mrs. Pelino would have died of pneumonia."

"Do you think that was her desire?"

"Yes, sir."

Paul nodded toward Dr. Dawson and turned to the judge, "No more questions, Your Honor."

The DA strolled across the floor. "Dr. Dawson, you've had many discussions with family members over the years about Code status. What do you do when you disagree with their decision?"

"I try to help them understand the situation and answer their questions."

"What if they persist in a decision that you disagree with?"

"I abide by their wishes and continue the discussions."

The DA waited in silence for several seconds and then asked, "Have you ever discontinued life support on a patient against their wishes or that of their family?"

Dr. Dawson's eyes darted toward Kate, and he swallowed hard. The DA hit the core. In a muted tone, he uttered, "No."

"Would you ever condone the withdrawal of life support from a patient against the wishes of the patient or her family?"

"No."

"No more questions." She returned to her table.

Paul looked straight ahead. His mouth was dry, and he didn't want Kate to see him swallow hard.

He sifted through a few documents and then lifted his head to address Judge Perry. "I'd like to call Mrs. Francis McMillan to the stand."

Mrs. McMillan was about five feet, four inches tall and very slender. She walked with deliberate but sure steps. She wore trendy glasses and a bright blue dress. The bailiff swore her in, and she took her seat in the witness stand.

Paul began, "Please tell us your name."

"Francis McMillan."

"How did you know Mrs. Pelino?"

"We were friends for about 35 years. We traveled together and shared many interests."

"Did you ever discuss end-of-life issues?"

"Yes we did."

"How did those issues come up?"

"We talked about all kinds of things at our weekly knitting club, the Knit-Wits." She paused and smiled. "In the past year, we lost two other friends, and their deaths motivated us to discuss these issues."

"Please explain."

"Both of these women, like Maria, had long, drawn-out periods of suffering before they finally died. Some of the women in our group had the opinion that they would rather not be kept alive under conditions like those.

"Others said they would rather live as long as possible with the hope that they would recover. They each had a friend with a miraculous recovery or they had seen one on television."

"How many times did you discuss these issues?"

"Several times over six months." Mrs. McMillan's eyes lit up and she said, "And let me tell you, these women don't just discuss things. They debate and argue like a bunch of attorneys."

"Did Mrs. Pelino participate in the debates?"

"Oh yes." A big smile broke across her face. "She was always in the middle of every debate. She loved the battle."

"What was her opinion?"

"She said it many times. The gist of it was something like, 'I would rather live well, than live long.' She always took the position that she would not want to be placed on machines to prolong her life."

"Did Maria ever talk about obtaining a Living Will or any other documents to address her end-of-life wishes?"

Mrs. McMillan sat silently and dropped her head. "She talked about getting that done, but she didn't. I'm embarrassed to say that none of us did despite all the debate and discussion. I guess we thought we'd get around to it later.

"Now we have our Living Will, power of attorney for health care, and Code status established."

"What encouraged you to proceed?"

"Maria's suffering. We watched her suffer through this misery against her wishes. That got us moving. We're making sure that doesn't happen to any of us.

"There are still a few in that group who expect a miracle, so they've made no changes. I don't agree with them, but I respect the fact that they thought it through and took a position."

"Did Maria Pelino want to live on a ventilator?"

"Absolutely not."

"I have no more questions. Thank you, Mrs. McMillan."

The DA did not arise from her chair. "I have no questions."

While Paul watched Mrs. McMillan return to her seat, he glanced at Kate out of the corner of his eye. Kate thought she detected the most subtle hint of a smirk on Paul's face, and then he said, "I call Dr. Jack Gerard to return to the stand."

39

Jack was leaning back and yawning when he heard his name. He jolted forward and stared at the DA. She nodded with what looked like discreet confidence and motioned toward the stand with a miniscule bob of her head. Jack breathed easier.

He stood, tightened his bright yellow tie, buttoned his jacket, adjusted his professionally styled hair with a swipe of his hand, and strolled to the stand. Each step seemed more confident than the last. He even winked at the CNN reporter on his way to the stand.

Paul wasted no time. "Dr. Gerard, please describe your working relationship with Dr. Simon."

"Dr. Simon was an intern at Mercy, and I am a senior resident." Kate detected his subtle emphasis on the words "was" and "am," as he stole a glance her way. "We both worked under the supervision of an attending physician, but I am responsible for the management and education of interns like Dr. Simon. We worked together to care for patients."

"Please describe the relationship Dr. Simon had with Mrs. Pelino."

"Dr. Simon had an emotional attachment to the patient and spent a lot of time with her."

"Please explain this 'emotional attachment.'"

Jack remained confident. "Dr. Simon spent numerous hours at the patient's bedside and attended to her needs…almost obsessively."

"Obsessively?" Paul raised his eyebrows and tilted his head.

"She visited the patient before rounds and examined her. She wrote orders to attend to matters and then returned after our rounds. She checked in late every afternoon, too.

"One night when I was on call, I found Dr. Simon at the patient's bedside holding her hand and talking to her. She was emotionally involved with this patient." Jack spewed with supremacy.

"Was Dr. Simon's care inappropriate?" Paul's voice lifted.

"She was too emotionally attached to the patient. I'd say it was inappropriate. Look how it ended," he said with disgust.

Kate stared at Jack. Her jaw clenched and she shook her head. She still could not deal with Jack as the hero doctor. Kate's stomach lurched.

With a deadpan expression and monotone, Paul asked, "How would you say your philosophy of patient care differed from Dr. Simon's?"

"First of all, I have two more years of patient care experience to inform my decisions. I provide good patient care and don't allow the emotions of a case to cloud my thinking."

In the exact same tone and sequence, Paul repeated, "You don't allow your emotions to cloud your thinking." He paused and then asked, "Are you a compassionate physician?"

Jack fidgeted and straightened in his seat. "I treat people properly," he said, sounding less certain.

Paul turned toward Jack and stared silently for several seconds with his arms crossed. Then he demanded, "Have you ever referred to one of your patients as a 'crack whore'?"

The words hit Jack like an uppercut. He wobbled and looked toward the DA. She took a deep breath, as her eyes darted away from Jack.

Jack sat stunned for several seconds, weighing his options. Finally he whispered, "I don't remember." He looked away from Paul.

Paul moved as close as possible and said, "Dr. Gerard, I remind you that you are under oath, and we are prepared to call other hospital staff to clarify this matter."

Jack froze. He enjoyed creating terror, but now he faced it. His media image was falling like a house of cards. One phrase was all it took to destroy Jack's image—crack whore. Finally he said, "I've used that term before."

"Did you ever use the term 'crack whore' to refer to one of the patients that you and Dr. Simon helped care for?"

Jack sighed. "Yes."

Murmurs filled the room, as several reporters scribbled notes. Judge Perry glared over his spectacles, and the rumble subsided as quickly as it had begun.

"Do you remember the conflict you and Dr. Simon had over the treatment of that patient?"

"Vaguely," Jack said. He still would not look at Paul.

"Please recall what you can."

"Dr. Simon wanted to delay the patient's hospital discharge to arrange for social services."

"Did you object to Dr. Simon's actions?"

"I didn't agree with the time she expended on the case," Jack said, as his face tightened.

"Do you remember what Dr. Simon did?"

"I believe she arranged for substance abuse treatment before the patient was discharged."

Paul asked, "What nickname did you conjure up for Dr. Simon?"

"I called her Dr. DoGood a few times. It was all in good fun. A nickname, you know," Jack pleaded.

"Dr. DoGood. How did you come up with that?" Paul quizzed.

"Like I said, Dr. Simon's approach is different than mine. She's more emotionally involved with patients and attentive to social concerns. That's why I called her Dr. DoGood."

Paul's jaw stiffened and he asked, "Did you ever mock her with the title, Dr. DoGood?"

Jack shifted again. He knew there were too many witnesses to his slander against Kate, so finally he mumbled, "I probably did."

"Did you assign most patients with difficult social issues, such as substance abuse and homelessness, to Dr. Simon?"

"She seemed to enjoy those cases, so I assigned them to her." Jack struggled to regain poise.

"Did she complain about taking care of these patients?"

"Not that I remember."

Paul strolled away from the stand but then spun back. "So you called her Dr. DoGood because of her compassion and concern for social issues. Her kindness stands in stark contrast to your cruel, callous heart. I'll take her as my doctor over you any day," Paul thundered.

The DA was so shocked by the exchange that she failed to object. Reporters wrote relentlessly, recording these revelations of Jack's character.

"No more questions, Your Honor." Paul shook his head with disgust as he walked back.

The DA collected her thoughts and conferred with her assistant. The damage was done. She stood and said, "No questions for Dr. Gerard."

Jack finally arose. Sweat beaded on his forehead, and his face was pale. He stumbled toward his seat like a punch-drunk fighter. The once-friendly CNN reporter refused to look at Jack as he returned. Jack bolted to the bathroom where he emptied his stomach.

40

As Kate watched Jack stumble out of the courtroom, her eyes met Paul's, and she struggled to restrain a grin. She knew who was up next. Paul turned toward the judge and said, "In light of Dr. Gerard's testimony, I would like to re-call Dr. Kate Simon."

Her shoulders and chest lifted with a deep inspiration; she closed her eyes for a few seconds as she stood. Every eye traced her movements toward the stand.

"Was Dr. Gerard's nickname, Dr. DoGood, a common title for you?"

"He used that title whenever our supervising physician was not around. He knew the attending would not approve."

"Describe your relationship with Dr. Gerard."

"It was strained because we treated people much differently. Dr. Gerard treated people as an organism with a disease, and I tried to treat them as humans. We disagreed mostly over treatment of poor people and drug abusers. He treats these people with contempt, and he hated me because I cared for these people with compassion."

"Can you give an example?"

"We had a young woman with chest pain due to use of crack cocaine. She was a prostitute. I found out that she was abandoned by her family when she was 12 and moved from family to family as a teenager. She ended up on the streets, and a pimp picked her up.

"From that time, prostitution was all she knew, but she confided in me that she wanted out of it and wanted help getting off crack. I proposed that we help her get into drug rehab. Dr. Gerard was not happy with the extra effort these arrangements took, and that's when he started calling me Dr. DoGood. From that point forward our relationship deteriorated."

"Why did it deteriorate?"

"Dr. Gerard would not relent from his view of these people, and I would not become nasty and cynical toward them. Every time I treated these people with dignity, he bristled. He controlled the patient mix of the interns, so Dr. Gerard began giving me only the difficult social problems. It was okay by me on one hand, but on the other, he deprived me of getting to work with a wider range of patients."

"Why didn't you report his behavior?"

"We had only been there for a few months, so I figured we'd be able to work it out. I've worked with cynics and sexists before, and I was not going to let him dominate me."

"Dr. Gerard critiqued you for being 'over-involved emotionally' with some of your patients. He pointed to the instance of you holding Mrs. Pelino's hand as an example. What's your reaction?"

"Dr. Gerard and I are polar opposites. He's aggravated by my care and concern for patients. My love for people underscores his callousness, and it torments him. I really cared about Mrs. Pelino, and I know what she told me. Her wishes were clear and I couldn't forget them. I suffered watching her suffer. That's why I was attentive to her.

"Living on a ventilator in an ICU is agonizing. Even though we sedate patients, they still suffer, so I wanted to do everything I could to relieve her pain."

Kate stopped and dropped her head. She swallowed hard and wiped her eye with the back of her hand. Silence filled the room.

"I sat at her bedside and held her hand because she relaxed when I talked to her, and at times, she gripped my hand." Kate looked at Paul through misty eyes. She bit her lip and continued through tears. "No one else sat with her and comforted her. Her son chose to keep her alive, but he never sat with her and held her hand. He did nothing to console her.

"I couldn't stand by like Dr. Gerard and watch someone suffer, when I knew I could provide comfort." Kate held back her sobs, but tears trickled.

Paul allowed Kate to collect herself and then asked, "You'd been in training for just a few months when this happened. How did you develop these strong opinions?"

"In those months, I watched many people suffer needlessly. Every day you can go through the halls of Mercy, or any hospital, and find elderly people who are suffering through their last days of life because they or their family have not discussed end-of-life decisions with a doctor. They come to the hospital, and we have no choice but do everything to keep them alive until we can establish Code status. In so many cases, we keep them alive, but we can't give them quality of life. It's horrible!" Kate couldn't believe her outburst but felt strengthened.

"What's makes it so bad for the patient?"

"Many of our interventions are painful and offer little chance of restoring a person to health. For example, in the first month of my internship, I was so enthusiastic about resuscitating patients—"

Paul interrupted. "Please explain 'resuscitating.'"

"When a patient's heart stops or they stop breathing, we try to revive them. We use CPR, which means we press heavily on the chest. We press hard enough to compress the heart through the chest and circulate blood. Then we insert a tube into the windpipe and provide breaths with a bag device. We follow protocols using electrical shocks and medications in attempts to restore circulation."

"Okay, please resume your account."

"I was excited about resuscitation because we saved a young guy's life one night, but later I saw the other side of resuscitation. I was called to Code an elderly woman. I can still see her frail body, lifeless and peaceful on the bed until we started...I started chest compressions."

Kate stopped. Her mouth was suddenly dry. She swallowed hard, remembering the feeling of that woman's disintegrating sternum. She resumed, "I started chest compressions, and I broke her breast bone and ribs. With every compression, I felt bones crumble. I'll never forget it."

"What was the outcome of that resuscitation?"

"We revived her and put her in the ICU. Her outlook was terrible, and the family made a decision to stop care and let her die naturally. They changed her status to Do Not Resuscitate. It was tragic."

"Tragic?" quizzed Paul.

"Because Code status was not discussed before the lady died— the first time. We could have let her die in peace and not put her through the agony of resuscitation if only the Code status conversation would have occurred earlier."

"But what about hope for a longer life?"

"Dr. Dawson said it earlier. For elderly people with other illnesses, the chance of any quality of life after resuscitation is very low. About five percent.

The saddest part of the story is that most people don't have a clue about this well-documented fact. Research shows that most people over age 70 believe their chance of surviving resuscitation in a hospital and being discharged is about 50 percent. So their estimate is off by a factor of five to 10." Eyes were wide. Some jaws dropped.

Kate continued, "According to one study, people get their medical facts from television and end up thinking they have a decent chance of surviving resuscitation. The truth is that resuscitation of elderly people is practically futile."

"How did this impact your decision about Mrs. Pelino?"

"I was not about to let her go through that. She suffered enough." Kate's face froze.

"But Mrs. Pelino did receive resuscitation efforts before you declared her dead. Didn't she suffer through that?"

Kate's emotion evaporated. In a monotone she said, "I waited for several minutes before calling the Code to be sure she would not feel pain. She was dead when I called the Code."

"How long did you wait?"

"About 20 minutes."

"So for 20 minutes you sat at her bedside with the risk of being discovered, so she would not experience pain. What did you do during that time?"

"I held her hand and talked to her," Kate said as emotion flooded back. Those last minutes were impossible to forget. Kate sniffled, wiped her nose, and went on. "She was well sedated, but I spoke softly to her and stroked her hand and arm. She was tranquil in those last minutes. She died in peace and that's what she wanted." Kate hesitated and whispered again, "That's what she wanted."

Paul sighed. "Your Honor, I have no more questions." Paul glanced at the jurors. They sat transfixed by emotion—Kate's and theirs. He wondered if they could forgive her.

Eager to abate the emotion and intensifying empathy toward Dr. Simon, the DA jumped up and asked, "Dr. Simon, have you ever heard of a Messiah Complex?"

"Yes."

"A woman with a Messiah Complex believes herself to be a savior of a person or a group of people. She has an elevated view of herself and her opinions. I find no other motive in your case except for a Messiah Complex. In your eagerness to help a patient, you overstepped your authority. Do you believe you overstepped your authority?"

"I overstepped the authority of the State of Ohio." Before the DA could continue, Kate asked, "Do you think there is a higher authority?" She looked at the DA and then throughout the courtroom. She continued, "What about your conscience, your values, your god?"

The DA crossed her arms and said with a touch of sarcasm, "The authority you face today is the State of Ohio, and the charge is murder. Your conscience, your values, your god bear no weight in this court."

"I guess my values and conscience matter to me."

The DA lifted her eyebrows as a new thought emerged. "Are there other values that impacted your decision?"

Kate sat motionless while her thoughts raced. There was another reason, but she wondered if anyone would understand. Every eye converged on Kate. Her heart raced, and her eyes darted toward Paul. He knew nothing of this motive. Paul's furrowed brow and stern stare pleaded with her to be silent. She didn't want to let him down, but the truth mattered to Kate.

She was leaning back and her eyes were closed. She drew a deep breath and spoke clearly. "Toni Jackson."

The DA stood in silence and returned to her desk. She could not recall that name from the deposition.

Disbelief spread across Paul's face. He hadn't heard of Toni Jackson either.

Murmurings swelled in the courtroom as the spectators wondered about the identity of this mysterious Toni Jackson. Another suspect, a witness, or who? Paul glanced into the crowd. His gaze met the knowing eyes of Dr. Dawson, and Paul gulped.

Judge Perry scowled and slammed the gavel. "Order! Order!"

The DA looked perplexed but remained focused.

"What?" blasted the DA, shaking her head. "Or should I say, who?"

"Toni was another patient of mine. She was a 22-year-old woman who died because she couldn't afford a vial of insulin."

"What does that have to do with Mrs. Pelino's death?"

"You asked me if there were other values that impacted my decision. We can't forget Toni Jackson when we take care of patients like Mrs. Pelino."

The DA broke eye contact. Confusion was uncommon for her. She weighed her options, looked back at Kate, and asked, "Please help me understand what you're talking about."

"Here's the problem. People like Mrs. Pelino are ready to die, and yet we prolong their dying at great financial cost. Her hospitalization cost tens of thousands of dollars, and we were prepared to spend thousands more at a long-term acute-care hospital. And what would we accomplish for her? More misery.

"Then you have Toni Jackson, an uninsured single student, who dies because she was afraid to run up her hospital bill. That's not right! Do you see a problem with that?" Kate peered right through the DA into the courtroom.

The DA had never been cross-examined by a witness before, and she was dumbfounded. She returned to her desk, but then turned and fired, "So you killed Mrs. Pelino because she was a financial drain on society?"

"Mrs. Pelino died of natural causes just like she wanted to. Are we prepared to sit around and pretend that we have unlimited resources to plow into health care? Let's get real here. Are you ready to write a blank check for health care?"

The DA was silent so Kate went on.

"Only five percent of Medicare patients die each year, and still about 30 percent of Medicare expenditures go toward the last year of life. And half of that is spent in the last two months. That means 15 percent of all Medicare expenditures go into the last two months of life. In 2008, that was *$68 billion*. When you realize that a great deal of that care was unnecessary and unwanted, you begin to realize our system is broken."

"Do you have a bias against elderly people?"

"I love elderly people, like I did Mrs. Pelino, but our health care finances are running dry, and we face crucial decisions."

The DA wanted to give Kate some rope and hoped she would hang herself, so she encouraged the denunciation. "And what solutions would you offer?"

Kate pressed on. "If elderly patients knew the realities of the health care system and talked about the issues with their doctors, many would decline futile measures like resuscitation and other futile treatments.

"The answer is not rules or rationing of health care, but discussion! Patients and families can learn the facts, and doctors can advise them. Rigid rules cannot accommodate people's complex situations and beliefs. Discussions need to occur before the end is near, so patients, doctors, and families understand each other."

Kate hesitated, wondering whether she should stop. The DA nodded toward her, leaving more slack in the rope.

"I've had a lot of time to think about this while sitting in that cell. There are other things that the government could do. They could pay doctors adequately to initiate these difficult conversations. A conversation like that takes time and energy to organize and execute. Medicare's payment to primary care doctors is dismal. It barely covers their costs to have the conversation.

"Then we sit here and wonder why the doctors don't do it often enough." Kate spit out the final words in disgust. "Medicare won't pay a doctor to have a conversation about Code status even though it could save thousands of people from the agony of unwanted, painful procedures like resuscitation. Then they turn around and pay thousands for futile health care on people who are suffering and can't get well.

"I've had a lot of time to look into this, and the way our system treats primary care physicians is pitiful. Medicare pays a doctor according to the level of service and time spent face-to-face with a patient. Doctors receive about $90 for a 25-minute visit and around $120 for 40 to 70 minutes. That's what they receive to cover all the expenses of running an office and their salary. Besides that, they receive no compensation for services they provide through phone conversations or other non-face-to-face interactions like email. Most patients and family members expect doctors to discuss matters on the phone and don't realize that Medicare refuses payment for those services. With that level of reimbursement, a doctor can barely cover his or her overhead, let alone make much profit." Kate riveted her eyes on the DA. "Would *you* work for that?"

All eyes in the courtroom were fixed on Kate. The DA remained silent.

Kate paused and decided to go on. "Another problem is the Living Will. In Ohio and many other states, people feel secure if they have a Living Will. It helps sometimes, but the Ohio Living Will does not address Code status. It only applies to situations where a patient is terminally ill or in a permanently unconscious state. What we need is a Living Will that gives people the option, Do Not Resuscitate. At least people need to know that Living Wills don't address Code status in most situations, so they can take that up with their physician.

"If these measures were in place, people could die in peace and with dignity before they end up in one of these terrible, terminal, death-prolonging conditions. Let's stop measuring the quality of medical care based on the number of hours a person lives. We need to start helping people die well." Kate finished in a flurry. Did she hang herself? They would know shortly.

The DA looked satisfied. "No more questions." Paul looked terrified.

Their closing arguments would conclude the trial.

After a short recess, the courtroom filled for closing arguments. The DA presented the State's case first. She began, "Ladies and gentlemen of the jury, from the beginning, one thing has been absolutely clear. Dr. Kate Simon caused Maria Pelino's death. No one in this courtroom denies that fact.

"Maria Pelino died that night because Dr. Simon decided it was time for her to die. The laws of this nation and state are written to protect citizens against actions like hers. Dr. Simon committed premeditated murder that night.

"She painstakingly planned the crime. She waited for the right moment to commit it and carried it out as planned. She accomplished her goal. She ended Maria Pelino's life. She murdered Mrs. Pelino and getting caught is her only regret.

"Her defense glorified her as a hero who acted in the patient's best interest. She wants you to believe that she is the champion of the sick and caretaker of the afflicted.

"Dr. Simon said she believed she was acting in Mrs. Pelino's best interest, but she murdered her. She acted against the clearly expressed and legally protected wishes of the patient's next of kin. Dr. Simon imposed her will and killed Mrs. Pelino. She is no different than a vigilante on the streets. Some lionize a vigilante, but civilized society cannot tolerate vigilante behavior. We cannot allow people, and particularly doctors, to take human life into their hands.

"Dr. Simon admits her mistakes. She says her mistake was her failure to document her conversation. The horror arose when she followed that mistake with a terrible crime.

"All of us make mistakes. Most of us have made another mistake to cover the first one, but sooner or later the string of mistakes must end.

"You cannot allow this series of mistakes to continue."

The DA faced the jury and dropped her hands to her sides. Her voice was soft—barely audible to anyone but the judge and jurors. "What if that was your mother?" She paused as her eyes scanned every juror.

"What if you made a decision for *your* mother and a physician who *you* trusted violated that trust?

"How would you feel?"

She paused to allow her query to land. "Would you accept Dr. Simon's explanation?" Her intensity swelled.

"Would you stand by and permit Dr. Simon to impose her will on your loved one?" She stopped again. A few of the jurors shifted in their seats.

"You would not. Dr. Simon had no right to do what she did and now you can stand up for the rights of patients like Mrs. Pelino and their families by convicting Dr. Simon of aggravated murder.

"If you do not convict her, then you will send a message of tolerance and support to health care workers for vigilante health care. You will endorse the capricious use of their authority if you do not convict her.

"Dr. Simon made many mistakes, but the preeminent one was to play God. Her guilt is clear. You must convict her to protect this city and this country from criminals like her. She is a murderer with the readiness and drive to inflict her will on others—even at great personal risk.

"Dr. Simon is not a hero. She is a vigilante, and we do not tolerate vigilantes in this country. Convict her today and close the door on future outlandish abuses of power."

The DA walked back to her desk and closed her notebook, as she took her seat.

Paul stole one last glance at the scrawl on his yellow legal pad before he stood. Still looking down, he sipped some ice water. Paul had not only survived the shock of Kate's outburst, but he fashioned a demeanor that seemed surreal, almost tranquil. Paul's poise permeated the room. Even Kate felt at ease and her confidence revived.

The crowd heard every step, as he sauntered across the room. "Did your parents ever warn you with a saying like 'Never tell a lie,' or 'Never steal?'" He smiled as the jurors faces softened.

His tone was like a chat over coffee, and he detected a few nods of affirmation to his query. Paul continued, "We all know that it is wrong to lie and steal, but consider this. Is it always wrong to lie or steal?" Paul nailed "always."

He paused and repeated, "Is it always wrong to lie? Is it always wrong to steal? If you were poor and your children were starving, would it be right to steal food? If you were protecting a friend from an enemy, would it be wrong to lie to the enemy?

"Life is extremely complex, and at times, we must reconsider our basic thoughts about right and wrong. If I'm protecting a friend from a vicious enemy, then it is right to lie." Paul waited and lifted an eyebrow, giving time for the thought to sink in. "Yes, ladies and gentlemen, under special circumstances, it is right to lie. In other special circumstances, it is right to steal.

"This is true even though you've grown up thinking 'Never lie and never steal.' Sometimes protecting a friend outweighs telling the truth. Feeding a starving child trumps 'Don't steal.' We temper the absolute letter of the law with common sense.

"But today we are not talking about lying or stealing. We are talking about life and death. Is prolonging life to the greatest extent always in a person's best interest? Can you imagine instances where a shorter life would be a better life? Mrs. Pelino wanted to live a shorter life but only if it would be a better life. She did not want her death prolonged. The testimony of her friend of 35 years, Mrs. Francis McMillan, makes Mrs. Pelino's end-of-life thoughts perfectly clear.

"Mrs. Pelino's son, Thomas Pelino, acted to preserve his mother's life. Guilt drove his decisions, not concern for the good of his mother. He abandoned his mother years ago over money and emerged from the shadows to haunt her dying days with his tireless drive to keep her alive at all cost. She suffered every day, and he didn't even comfort her at her bedside. Only one person comforted her. The person who demonstrated deep care and concern for Mrs. Pelino, even love—is Dr. Kate Simon."

Paul drove his argument forward, and his tone intensified. "Dr. Kate Simon is on trial for aggravated murder. Have you beheld a calculating murderer over the past two days? Have you observed the mind and demeanor of a criminal?

"Dr. Simon is a compassionate, dynamic person who strives to care for people. In her, you see love—true and unselfish concern for other human beings. She moved to relieve Mrs. Pelino's agony at great personal risk. She risked her future. She risked her life.

"There are few doctors, few human beings that demonstrate heroism like this. You heard her speak and felt her compassion. Dr. Simon is not a murderer."

He paused and with full conviction concluded, "Affirm that today and allow this bright, young, caring physician's life to blossom. Her life is in your hands." Paul strolled back to the table.

Kate whispered, "You were awesome. I hope I didn't blow it."

Judge Perry instructed the jurors and asked them to start their deliberations at nine the next morning. Kate scanned their faces, knowing they would determine her destiny.

Judge Perry concluded, "Court will resume after the jury reaches a verdict. Court adjourned."

42

Kate returned down the long corridor to her cell, listening to the clanging of her chains. During dinner, the evening news flashed on the TV. Kate was the headliner again, and her fellow inmates cast admiring glances. They enjoyed the presence of celebrity. Kate hated the attention, but the short interview with Dr. Gerard made it worthwhile.

The TV reporter caught Jack as he emerged from the bathroom. Jack's hair was disheveled and his face was pale. The bright tie hung loosely and was spattered with chunks of vomit.

Unaware that the camera was running, Jack staggered down the hall when the reporter confronted him. His startled expression stood in stark contrast to his usual haughty manner. He tightened his tie and tried to pull himself together.

Kate laughed out loud with the other prisoners. The reporter looked at Jack with indignation and fired, "Do you have any other names for your patients, Doctor?"

Jack looked dazed. He looked around, mumbled, "No comment," and sprinted away into a media gauntlet. It looked like he had a long night ahead of him.

Conversations were quiet that evening. Even the convicts empathized with Kate. Many knew what it was like to face a jury and their future. Kate had been in her cell for about half an hour after dinner when the guard banged on the door. "Visitor, Simon. Let's go."

Kate jumped up and draped a sweatshirt over her prison garb. They hustled to the visitation room. Several of the cubicles were full, and the guard pointed her toward number five. Kate saw Meg's red eyes as she rounded the corner.

Kate dropped her head and said, "Sorry, Meg. I blew it today."

"What do you mean?"

"I didn't need to get into medical costs and Toni Jackson. It's all true, but I'm sure it didn't help my case."

"Why did you bring it up?"

Kate shrugged and said, "She asked me if there were other factors that affected my decision about Mrs. Pelino. I thought people needed to know the whole story."

They discussed Kate's testimony at length. The tone lightened as they remembered Jack's spectacle on the stand that day.

Meg concluded, "I don't think your testimony hurt your case. You were honest and everyone could see that. Your lawyer did a fantastic job."

Their eyes met and Kate said, "You know, Meg, there's a good chance I'm gonna lose."

Meg bit her lip and remained silent. Then she nodded in agreement ever so slightly.

"I've been thinking about the future," Kate said, hesitating again. "I've had lots of time to think lately, and I've decided that no matter what, I won't quit."

"Quit?" Meg asked with surprise.

"No matter what happens, I can't stop trying to help people. It's who we are, Meg. I'm not going to get bitter and quit."

She gazed off briefly, and when she returned, a tear was rolling down her face. "I would miss being a doctor so badly. But it's not over, Meg."

Just then the guard returned and said, "Time's up, Simon."

Kate looked up and said, "Thanks for coming by, Meg. I'll see you tomorrow."

Meg wiped her eyes and forced a smile as they parted.

Not long after lunch the next day, the guard startled Kate, rapping on her door. Her shrill voice jolted Kate back to reality: "They have your verdict, Simon. Let's go."

She hurried to her feet, and the guard placed the shackles on her wrists and ankles. Every eye followed Kate as she wound through the cell block. Kate's footsteps echoed down the long corridor between jail and courthouse.

She entered the jammed courtroom. Scanning the crowd, she saw her friends, including Dr. Dawson, Meg, and many others. She knew how hard it must have been for Dr. Dawson to say the things he said. She had no animosity toward him. Jack's seat was empty. She was glad to see Paul, who'd become a friend and colleague during this nightmare. They sat at the defense table awaiting Judge Perry.

He entered and the jury followed. Every eye in the courtroom fixed on the jurors. Their unread decision was Kate's life. Judge Perry called the court to order and turned to the foreman. "Have you reached a verdict, sir."

The foreman rose slowly, and his gaze did not depart from the judge. "Yes, Your Honor. We find the defendant guilty of aggravated murder." Most of the jury members dropped their heads. None looked Kate's way.

Mr. Pelino smiled and shook the DA's hand. No one cheered. The media scattered, taking up strategic positions. Some waited for Thomas Pelino and the DA. Others lingered, awaiting Kate's entourage, who'd been battered like they received news of a tragic death.

Meg's head was in her hands, and her shoulders trembled as the tears poured forth. Dr. Dawson, who was seated next to Meg, leaned forward so that he was immediately next to her. He put his hand on her shoulder but said nothing. He had a look of agony and bewilderment.

Kate covered her head with both arms and sobbed. Paul slipped his arm around her shoulders and held her tight.

Paul looked up at Judge Perry and asked, "Your Honor, may we have a few minutes before Dr. Simon is taken away?"

"You may have five minutes," said the Judge.

Paul continued to console Kate as the minutes flew by. Grieving filled the room. Paul leaned down and said, "It's time to go, Kate."

She stood and looked at Meg and her friends. She couldn't believe what she'd put them through. Dr. Dawson squeezed through the crowd, bringing him within earshot of Kate as she was leaving. He asked, "Kate, may I visit you?"

She could only nod yes, but his act of kindness provided comfort that she had not felt for a long, long time.

43

Kate was deep in thought and flinched when the guard pounded on her door. "You have a visitor, Simon." Kate looked into a small mirror and hustled to brush her hair and get ready for the visit. She wondered who the visitor might be and hoped it was Dr. Dawson.

When she entered the cubicle, she was relieved to see Dr. Dawson, but she had never seen this look of apprehension on his face.

Kate sat down and Dr. Dawson said, "Kate, I'm so sorry. I feel like I let you down. I knew you were in agony, as Mrs. Pelino was lingering, and I didn't talk to you about it. I failed you."

"Dr. Dawson, this is my fault, not yours. How could you ever expect one of your residents to do this?"

"I didn't expect this, but I still believe I could have done more to help you. For that, please forgive me."

It was the last thing Kate expected to hear. She smiled. "I forgive you."

Dr. Dawson took a deep breath. His expression softened. It seemed to Kate that a huge burden had been lifted from his shoulders. "Thanks, Kate. Is there anything I can do for you now?"

"I've been thinking about what I'm going to do in here. Remember, a life sentence is mandatory, and that's a long time."

Dr. Dawson looked down and shook his head. "Yes, I remember."

"I guess I'll need some very long-term goals," Kate said and laughed.

She continued, "There are a few things that I could do here in prison. I might be able to help educate other prisoners. Maybe they would let me start a medical technician training program or something like that."

"I'm glad that you're not giving up. I'll do whatever I can to help you succeed."

"Thanks, Dr. Dawson. After that trial, I'm more convinced than ever about the need to get people educated about end-of-life issues, too. I may be able to do some of that from this side of the wall."

"You could become an expert in the field even in here. I'm willing to keep you supplied with journals and books. We may even be able to collaborate on research. You could formulate the ideas and analyze the data, and I could get the data for you. I'm sure I can recruit residents to help."

Kate's spirits lifted with the hope of doing something productive. She asked, "When do you think you can deliver the first stack of books?"

Epilogue

Eight years later, the northwest doors to the Oval Office swung open, and a party of legislators strolled through. They gathered around the President's desk to witness the signing of a bill. The sponsor of the bill, Senator Harold Stowe from Ohio, presented the legislation. It was labeled *Ending Life with Compassion Act* and included provisions for physician and public education about end-of-life issues.

It created a standardized Living Will that included designations for DNR and funding for a national computer registry of all Medicare patients' Code status.

The bill also amended Medicare, so physicians would be properly reimbursed for having end-of-life discussions.

It sailed through Congress with bipartisan support because the points were simple and practical, to say nothing of the billions of precious health care dollars to be saved by not providing futile and unwanted care. Those dollars would be available to care for the uninsured of all ages. The bill was touted as a service to the elderly and to society.

The President signed the bill, glanced up at Senator Stowe with a grin, and said, "That's a feather in your cap, Harry." Senator Stowe puffed his chest, but before he could manage a "thank you," another Senator interrupted, "You know, sir, the real sponsor is a little woman in an Ohio prison."

Senator Stowe nodded his head in agreement. "Most of the ideas came from her," he said with some reluctance.

The President pushed the bill to the corner of the desk, turned to his Chief of Staff, and said, "I'd like to know more about that prisoner."

Source Notes

16   See appendix *Facts About Resuscitation*

      Kerin Jones. "The Knowledge And Perceptions of Medical
      Personnel Relating To Outcome After Cardiac Arrest,"
      Resuscitation, 2006; Vol. 69, No. 2. pp. 235-239.

17   Susan J. Diem. "Cardiopulmonary Resuscitation on
      Television—Miracles and Misinformation," *N Engl J Med.*
      1996, Vol. 334, No. 24, pp.1578-1582.

41   Samuel Zuvekas. "Prescription Drugs and the Changing
      Concentration of Health Care Expenditures," *Health Affairs.*
      2007, Vol. 26, No. 1, pp. 249-257.

46   Kaiser Health Tracking Poll: October 2008. "Nearly half (47
      percent) of the public reports someone in their family skipping
      pills, postponing or cutting back on medical care they said they
      needed in the past year due to the cost of care. For example,
      just over one-third say they or a family member put off or
      postponed needed care and three in 10 say they skipped a
      recommended test or treatment — increases of seven
      percentage points from last April's tracking poll which asks the
      same question."
      <www.kff.org/kaiserpolls/h08_posr102108pkg.cfm>.

58   Payment as of January 2009 in Columbus, Ohio. Relative
      Weight 0.8696.

64   Donald Hoover. "Medical Expenditures During the Last Year
      of Life: Findings from the 1992-1996 Medicare Current
      Beneficiary Survey - Cost of Care," *Health Services Research J.*
      2002, Vol. 37, No. 6, pp.1625-1642.

95   Susan L. Mitchell. "Decisions to Forgo Hospitalization in
      Advanced Dementia: A Nationwide Study," *J Am Geriatric Soc.*
      2007, Vol. 55, pp.432-438.

141   Kamal Khalafi. "Avoiding the Futility of Resuscitation,"
      Resuscitation. 2001, Vol. 50, No. 2, pp. 161-166.

      Mohammad Saklayen. "In-Hospital Cardiopulmonary
      Resuscitation. Survival in One Hospital and Literature
      Review," *Medicine* (Baltimore). 1995, Vol. 74, No. 4, pp.163-75.

150   Susan J. Diem. "Cardiopulmonary Resuscitation on
      Television—Miracles and Misinformation," *N Engl J Med*.
      1996, Vol. 334, No. 24, pp.1578-1582.

153   James D. Lubitz. "Trends in Medicare Payments in the Last
      Year of Life," *N Engl J Med*. 1993, Vol. 328, No. 15, pp.1092-
      1096.

      Total Medicare Budget, February 5, 2007 per HHS was $454
      billion.

154   These figures are for 2009: 25-minute office visit is billed with
      code 99214-$89.88; 40 minutes to 70 minutes 99215-$121.83.
      At 70 minutes, a doctor can add an additional prolonged
      service code 99354 - $90.80 for an additional hour.

Afterword

What can be done to remedy this costly end-of-life disaster of prolonged dying? We are not powerless against this wave of hardship.

The solution is not rules or rationing of health care resources, but education. That is the purpose of this book. I hope you will read through this appendix to get more facts and suggestions.

When physicians, patients, and their loved ones understand and discuss the facts about end-of-life care, they make good medical decisions. In most situations, good medical decisions are good financial decisions. Given the opportunity, most people would not choose a prolonged painful death. Instead, they would choose a natural, dignified death.

Public policy makers should read this carefully and digest the facts. The rest of us can contact our legislators to encourage them to act. We have no hope of health care reform if we neglect this issue. End-of-life care simply consumes too many resources and will continue to grow without changes.

I do not advocate physician-assisted suicide. I believe we should allow people to die naturally, *if they choose*, and not face prolonged dying. Do yourself, your loved ones, and our society a favor—investigate these issues and obtain a Living Will and Durable Power of Attorney for Health Care, and decide on Code status as soon as possible.

Jeff Gordon, M.D.
Grant Medical Center
Columbus, Ohio

Appendix: Facts and Opinions

Contents

Get current resources and ideas at:

End of Life Education
www.eoleducation.org

Conversations and Decisions Needed

A Death Prolonged has probably answered some questions and raised others. My goal is to encourage more dialogue about these crucial issues, so every person can make well-informed end-of-life decisions. Ultimately, I hope we will be able to work toward legislative changes that will promote these discussions.

Change is possible, and the prospect of a tremendously positive outcome is truly exciting. We could help millions of people make informed end-of-life decisions that would avoid prolonged dying and in the process save billions of precious health care dollars. Let's explore what you can do to advocate for change.

For Everyone

Most importantly, talk about the issue. Death needs to come into public discussion. Our population is aging, and every year we delay this discussion, we will witness more and more needless suffering and expanding health care spending.

- ☐ Discuss the issues with friends and consider a book club to talk about *A Death Prolonged.*

- ☐ Write down your personal end-of-life wishes and discuss them with your family, friends, and physician.

- ☐ Talk to your attorney and create a Living Will and a Durable Power of Attorney for Health Care. Include Code status designations, if possible.

- ☐ Whether you have a Living Will or not, discuss Code status with your physician, and every time you visit a hospital, be sure your physicians know your wishes.

- ☐ Nursing home residents need to know that they have the option of Do Not Resuscitate with Comfort Care only. The patient (or designated decision maker) may also designate Do Not Hospitalize, which allows the patient to remain under Comfort Care in the nursing home without being moved to a hospital or emergency room. This is a wise choice for many elderly patients because in their last months of life additional measures only prolong their dying and cause unnecessary suffering.

- ☐ Web resources: **www.eoleducation.org**
  End of Life/Palliative Education Resource Center:
  www.eperc.mcw.edu

The American Thoracic Society:
www.thoracic.org/sections/clinical-information/critical-care/patient-information/index.html

Physicians

- ☐ Develop your own style for raising end-of-life issues with your patients. The approaches depicted by characters in *A Death Prolonged* are suggestions you could imitate. Always include the facts about resuscitation survival rates.
- ☐ Include the facts about resuscitation to help objectify decisions.
- ☐ Provide background reading to prepare patients for end-of-life discussions. You may visit **www.eoleducation.org** or **www.eperc.mcw.edu** to obtain free patient education materials.
- ☐ Take time to discuss the issues with your patients and document their decisions.

Pastors

- ☐ Get educated on the facts of end-of-life care.
- ☐ During hospital visits, ask patients if they have discussed Code status and be sure they also understand it. Be sure they understand that the Living Will does not usually address Code status.
- ☐ In your communication and teaching work, advocate for awareness on these issues and point out that most people are misinformed on the facts about end-of-life care.

Attorneys and Financial Planners

- ☐ Encourage your clients to obtain a Living Will and a Durable Power of Attorney for Health Care. Designate Code status if possible.
- ☐ Encourage your clients to discuss Code status with their physicians and inform them that most Living Wills do not address Code status.
- ☐ Advocate for changes in Living Will legislation to address Code status.
- ☐ Encourage clients to inform their physician regarding their end-of-life decisions.
- ☐ Advocate for educational efforts at the national and state levels to improve understanding of these issues in the legal community.

Policy Makers

☐ Advocate for standard education materials to inform patients and physicians of the risks and benefits of resuscitation.

☐ Advocate that Medicare reimburse primary care physicians for end-of-life discussions based on a procedure code that is different than an office visit. The level of reimbursement should correlate with time spent and should provide generous payment for this difficult task. Compare payment for primary care to specialty care, such as radiology and cardiology, to help guide reimbursement (see section *How is Physician Reimbursement Set?* later in the appendix).

☐ Develop a nationwide database for end-of-life decisions that medical personnel could quickly access. This would prevent mistaken resuscitation of patients when they arrest outside the hospital or when they move from one institution to another. It would also save health care providers a great amount of time and effort in trying to determine Code status. We should make every effort to honor end-of-life wishes with a system such as this. Studies show that many patients are resuscitated against their stated wishes because medical personnel do not have access to their documented decisions.

☐ Provide a nationally standardized Living Will that includes designation for Code status.

☐ Develop a national education program to intervene against the misinformation that television has created about the success rates of resuscitation. Remember, based on television, most elderly people believe they have about a 50 percent chance of being successfully resuscitated when the truth is much, much lower (see *The Facts About Resuscitation*, next section of the appendix). If other medical interventions were this ineffective, the public would know about it, and most people would refuse such futile interventions.

The Facts about Resuscitation

"While most people believe that CPR works 60-85% of the time, in fact the actual survival to hospital discharge is more like 10-15% for all patients and less than 5% for the elderly and those with serious illnesses."

Charles F. von Gunten, MD PhD and David E. Weissman, MD presented this summary. Find more at:

End of Life/Palliative Education Resource Center (EPERC)
www.eperc.mcw.edu/fastFact/ff_024.htm
www.eperc.mcw.edu/fastFact/ff_023.htm

Summary of the medical literature on resuscitation:

Interpreting the data on in-hospital resuscitation is not easy because some studies include both respiratory and cardiac arrests. Resuscitation rates are always better when respiratory arrests are included (CPR is not needed in a pure respiratory arrest). These studies look at various end-points to evaluate the effectiveness of resuscitation including return of spontaneous circulation (ROSC), 24-hour survival, three-month survival, and one-year survival. Most studies emphasize short-term results, and few look at one-year survival. A representative study showed immediate resuscitation rates of 44% with 15% survival to discharge, but only a 5% one year survival.[1] Another study showed 34.5% recovered from arrest, 12% left the hospital, and only 8.5% survived six weeks.[2]

When we exclude respiratory arrest (only including cardiac arrest requiring CPR) and look at patients over age 70, survival to discharge is predominantly less than 10% with a few studies showing higher survival rates.

Survival rates vary widely based on factors that I will discuss below. For example, in one study of resuscitation for cardiac arrest of patients over age 70, there were no survivors to discharge.[3] Another

---

[1] Mohammad Saklayen. "In-hospital Cardiopulmonary Resuscitation: Survival in 1 Hospital and Literature Review," *Medicine* (Baltimore). 1995, Vol. 74, No. 4, pp.163-175.

[2] Kamal Khalafi. "Avoiding the Futility of Resuscitation," *Resuscitation*. 2001, Vol. 50, No. 2, pp.161-166.

[3] G. E. Taffet. "In-hospital Cardiopulmonary Resuscitation," *JAMA*. 1988, Vol. 260, No. 14, pp. 2069-2072.

Canadian study found a 1% survival to discharge for patients that suffered an unwitnessed cardiac arrest in the hospital.[4] Therefore, we need to know what factors lead to significant success with resuscitation vs. factors that predict a poor outcome.

Factors Impacting Outcomes for In-hospital Cardiac Arrests

Positive Predictors	Negative Predictors
Hospital Setting: - Operating Room - Cardiac Catheterization Lab - Emergency Room - Coronary Care Unit	Hospital Location - General Medical/Surgical Unit - Intensive Care Unit
Witnessed arrest	Unwitnessed arrest
Ventricular fibrillation as initial rhythm	Pneumonia
Respiratory arrest (no CPR)	Older age
Short duration of CPR	Other medical conditions
	Initial rhythm: pulseless electrical activity or asystole
	Previous CPR

5,6,7,8,9

These studies focus on in-hospital resuscitation. Out-of-hospital resuscitation rates are significantly lower.

The other factor to consider is that about 40% of those resuscitated in one study had a significant neurological injury.[10]

Based on these data, who should consider requesting DNR?

This is a deeply personal decision and one that should be discussed carefully among family members and with one's personal

---

[4] Peter Brindley. "Predictors of Survival Following In-Hospital Adult Cardiopulmonary Resuscitation," *Can Med Ass J.* August 20, 2002, Vol. 4, p. 167.

[5] Maria Ann Peberdy. "Survival from In-Hospital Cardiac Arrest During Nights and Weekends," *JAMA.* 2008, Vol. 299, No. 7, pp.785-792.

[6] Brindley.

[7] Saklayen.

[8] S. Danciu. "A Predictive Model For Survival After In-Hospital Cardiopulmonary Arrest," *Resuscitation.* 2004, Vol. 62, No. 1, pp. 35-42.

[9] Khalafi.

[10] Danciu.

physician. I recommend that you take this list to your physician and ask him or her to review your condition in view of these predictors. You should also consider these factors when being admitted to a hospital.

If you are admitted with a heart attack or heart rhythm problem, you will have the best chance of surviving resuscitation.

If you decide in favor of DNR, most hospitals have a policy of revoking the DNR during surgery or a cardiac catheterization since resuscitation rates are very high and you would be in a highly monitored environment. Discuss all these issues with your physicians.

Misinformation about resuscitation among physicians and the public:

Patients and physicians are unaware of the relative futility of cardiac resuscitation. This needs to change to enable patients to make informed decisions about end-of-life care.

Elderly Patients:

"An oral standardized survey was administered to 100 patients aged 70 years or older. Patients were randomly selected from the emergency department, internal medicine clinic, and general medical wards at one urban medical center."

Results: "Most respondents (81%) believed that their chance of surviving inpatient CPR and leaving the hospital was 50% or better, and 23% of those respondents believed that their chance was 90% or better."[11]

Physicians:

Most physicians do not know the success rate of in-hospital resuscitation.

Accurate in-hospital cardiac arrest estimates [% (95% CI)] of survival were provided by 51.1% (36.8-63.4%), 47.3% (35.9-58.7%), and 36.7% (23.2-50.2%) of students, residents, and attending physicians, respectively.[12]

Education Required:

Physicians and the general public need to know the facts about end-of-life care. They need to have a much better understanding of the success rates of resuscitation, so they can make informed decisions.

The Department of Health and Human Services could undertake an educational campaign targeting physicians on one hand and the public on the other.

---

[11] Derrick H. Adams. "How Misconceptions Among Elderly Patients Regarding Survival Outcomes of Inpatient Cardiopulmonary Resuscitation Affect Do-Not-Resuscitate Orders," *J Am Osteopathic Assoc*. 2006, Vol. 106, No. 7, pp.402-404.

[12] Kerin Jones. "The Knowledge and Perceptions of Medical Personnel Relating To Outcome After Cardiac Arrest," *Resuscitation*. 2006, Vol. 69, No. 2, pp. 235-239.

Living Will and a Durable Power of Attorney for Health Care

Both of these are important documents for everyone to have, but you must realize their limitations.

Living Will:
This is a legal document that expresses your desires for end-of-life care. In most states, these documents deal with end-of-life issues if you are in a "permanently unconscious state" or have a "terminal condition." In those cases, life support would be managed as you stipulate.

Unfortunately, in most states, the Living Will does NOT address Code status apart from the situations noted above. Therefore, someone who has a Living Will MUST ALSO DESIGNATE CODE STATUS to health care professionals, if he or she does not want to be resuscitated.

Durable Power of Attorney for Health Care:
This legal document gives authority to a designated person to make health care decisions on your behalf if you are unable.

Be sure to discuss your end-of-life wishes with the person you designate as your health care power of attorney.

Most attorneys can help you formulate these documents, and many hospitals provide these to patients.

State by state listing of Living Will laws:
The American Thoracic Society at:
www.thoracic.org/sections/clinical-information/critical-care/patient-information/making-decisions-about-the-end-of-life/description-of-different-advance-directives.html

Five Wishes
This document serves as a Living Will and a Power of Attorney for Health Care. You do not need an attorney to complete this form. It is a legal document in 40 states and can be obtained at: agingwithdignity.org or call 1-888-5-WISHES.

How is physician reimbursement set and what should change?
I argue in *A Death Prolonged* that reimbursement levels are not
adequate to promote physician discussion of end-of-life issues. In
this section, I describe the method used to determine payment levels,
and then I suggest a solution.

Payment rates are based on procedure codes, which are developed by
a committee composed of members of the physician community and
the insurance industry. Physician reimbursement is based on the
Resource Based Relative Value Scale (RBRVS), using these three
factors:
1. Physician Work
   - Physician time
   - Mental effort
   - Technical skill
   - Judgment
   - Stress
   - Amortization of physician's education
2. Practice Expense
3. Malpractice Expense

The factors of mental effort, judgment, and stress are extremely high
in end-of-life discussions, and therefore a high relative value should
be assigned to this type of effort. An end-of-life discussion is much
more stressful than a typical patient encounter and therefore should
have an independent code based on these criteria.

Proposed Solution:
- Assign procedure codes for end-of-life discussions.
- Physicians could qualify to bill Medicare, using these codes, after
  they complete a Continuing Medical Education program focused
  on end-of-life care. This education requirement would ensure
  that physicians provide accurate data to patients, allowing them
  to make informed end-of-life decisions.
- Patient education materials, developed nationally, could be
  provided to all physicians who request them and on the internet.
- Set the reimbursement level for these new procedure codes by
  comparing reimbursement for other procedures of comparable
  time, effort, and stress. Also compare reimbursement rates to
  procedures which are much less stressful, such as reading routine
  X-rays, removing ear wax, extracting a tooth, etc.
  Reimbursement for this extremely difficult and stressful

procedure should be higher than for procedures that require less time, effort, and stress.

Other Ideas for Saving Billions of Dollars

There are a few small, relatively inexpensive changes that could provide massive savings.

Shared Electronic Medical Records. We waste millions of dollars every day because we cannot easily share medical records between hospital systems. Case in point: Columbus, Ohio, has three major health systems, and when patients move from one to another, expensive tests are repeated.

For example, we frequently admit patients with chest or abdominal pain, who have been evaluated and treated in other Columbus hospitals. To obtain records, patients must complete a release-of-information form that is faxed to the other institution. That facility copies the medical records and faxes them back to us. This process takes so long that we are obliged to perform expensive diagnostic tests and often repeat the other hospital's evaluation, wasting thousands of dollars per patient. This scenario is common in every large city because many patients float from hospital to hospital.

The answer is easy. Share electronic medical records. We are unable to get this done due to concerns about privacy. With health care dollars in short supply, it's time to reconsider the privacy concerns and find ways to share medical records now. There are many scenarios hospitals could adopt to share information today without waiting for a county-, state-, or nation-wide system. Let's get creative and solve this problem. For instance, legislators may need to intervene to relax some of the extremely stringent privacy laws.

Bolster Reimbursement to Primary Care Physicians

I am not a primary care physician. I am a hospital-based internist. I argued for adequate reimbursement of primary care physicians for end-of-life discussions in *A Death Prolonged*. We need to get serious about improving payment to these doctors because we face a dramatic shortage of primary care physicians. Good primary care physicians can make wise choices and practice cost-effective health care.

A recent study published in the *Journal of the American Medical Association*[13] showed that only 2 percent of medical school graduates pursued specialty training in primary care internal medicine. That's down from 9% in 1990. Many students, whose average debt was $140,000, said that pay rate was a significant issue in their decision to not pursue primary care training.[14]

So far, the main intervention to increase interest in primary care has been to increase exposure to primary care during medical school. These interventions have not worked. The answer seems very simple: pay primary care physicians fairly. If we don't, we will not have doctors to serve our aging population.

---

[13] Mark H. Ebell. "Future Salary and US Residency Fill Rate Revisited," *JAMA*. 2008, Vol. 300, No. 10, pp.1131-1132.
[14] Karen E. Hauer. "Factors Associated With Medical Students' Career Choices Regarding Internal Medicine," *JAMA*. 2008, Vol. 300, No. 10, pp.1154-1164.

Bibliography

Adams, Derrick H. "How Misconceptions Among Elderly Patients Regarding Survival Outcomes of Inpatient Cardiopulmonary Resuscitation Affect Do-Not-Resuscitate Orders." *JAOA*, 2006; 106(7):402-404.

Brindley, Peter. "Predictors of Survival Following In-Hospital Adult Cardiopulmonary Resuscitation." *CMAJ*, August 20, 2002; 4:167.

Danciu, Soren C. "A Predictive Model For Survival After In-Hospital Cardiopulmonary Arrest." *Resuscitation*, 2004; 62(1):35-42.

Diem, Susan J. "Cardiopulmonary Resuscitation on Television — Miracles and Misinformation." *New Engl J Med*, June 13, 1996; 334(24):1578-1582.

Ebell, Mark H. "Future Salary and US Residency Fill Rate Revisited." *JAMA*, 2008; 300(10):1131-1132.

Hauer, Karen E. "Factors Associated With Medical Students' Career Choices Regarding Internal Medicine." *JAMA*, 2008; 300(10):1154-1164.

Hoover, Donald. "Medical Expenditures During the Last Year of Life: Findings from the 1992-1996 Medicare Current Beneficiary Survey—Cost of Care." *Health Services Research*, December 2002.

Jones, Kerin. "The Knowledge and Perceptions of Medical Personnel Relating to Outcome After Cardiac Arrest." *Resuscitation*, 2006; 69(2):235-239.

Kaiser Health Tracking Poll: October 2008, http://www.kff.org/kaiserpolls/h08_posr102108pkg.cfm.

Khalafi, Kamal. "Avoiding the Futility of Resuscitation." *Resuscitation*, 2001; 50(2):161-166.

Lubitz, James D. "Trends in Medicare Payments in the Last Year of Life." *New Engl J Med*, April 15, 1993; 328(15):1092-1096.

Mitchell, Susan L. "Decisions to Forgo Hospitalization in Advanced Dementia: A Nationwide Study." *JAGS*, 2007; 55:432-438.

Peberdy, Maria Ann. "Survival from In-Hospital Cardiac Arrest During Nights and Weekends." *JAMA*, 2008; 299(7):785-792.

Saklayen, Mohammad G. "In-Hospital Cardiopulmonary Resuscitation. Survival in One Hospital and Literature Review." *Medicine* (Baltimore), July 1995; 74(4):163-175.

Taffet, G. E. "In-hospital Cardiopulmonary Resuscitation." *JAMA*, 1988; 260(14): 2069-2072.

Wright, Alexi A. "Associations Between End-of-Life Discussions, Patient Mental Health, Medical Care Near Death, and Caregiver Bereavement Adjustment." *JAMA*, 2008; 300(14):1665-1673.

Zulekas, Samuel. "Prescription Drugs and the Changing Concentration of Health Care Expenditures." *Health Affairs*, 2007; 26(1):249-257.

Acknowledgments

This book has been a team effort, and therefore I have many people to thank. My friend, Dr. Pete Accetta, and I brainstormed for many months before I decided to write the story. He assisted and encouraged me throughout the process. My brother-in-law, Bob Stein, a communications professor and journalist, was my writing coach and executive editor. Dr. Warren Wheeler, my mentor in end-of-life issues and founder of hospice in central Ohio, provided much encouragement, and I thank him for instilling in me a profound appreciation for these matters.

Several people read the story and provided input on various versions and at various levels, and to all I am deeply indebted. They come from all walks of life. Physicians include Tim Benadum, MD, Jeff Barrows, DO, Mark Brownelle, MD, Charles Bush, MD, Phil Hawley, MD, Ben Humphrey, MD, Victoria Ruff, MD, Aroob Saleh, MD, Dhruti Suchak, MD, and Bruce Vanderhoff, MD.

Other health care professionals who helped me include John Allred, PhD, Charlette Gallagher-Allred, PhD, Ken Doka, PhD, Greg Rekos, DDS, Jennifer Rekos, DDS, Bruce Robinson, RN, Jill Steuer, PhD, RN, and Robert Wrenn, PhD.

Pastors Gary DeLashmutt, Lee Campbell and Dave Glover, who I serve with at Xenos Christian Fellowship, provided encouragement and feedback.

My friends Suzanne Accetta, Laura Avers, Lara Baker, Matt Boone, Roger Brucker, Helen Gordon, Jennifer Jones, Jennifer Hale, Tad Hale, Debbie Homan, Bill McKahan, Kim Miller, Joanne Rhodes, and Gene Whetzel all read the manuscript carefully and offered constructive ideas. Clay Cormany, PhD, made the final edits and to him I am deeply grateful.

My sister Lisa Gordon, a professor of English, helped immensely. My daughter Megan provided the perspective of a college student and my other children, Chris and Kate, put up with my talking about this book for the past year and encouraged me. My wife Laura has been there every step of the way.

These people sacrificed to help create this story because they believe there is hope for change. Each wants to see health care flourish in America and realizes that we must deal with end-of-life issues to have any hope for success.

I am most grateful to my Lord, Jesus Christ, who has changed my life and given me a heart of compassion. He's given me joy I did not expect or deserve, and a life's work that provides contentment.